Obesity

Recent Titles in the
CONTEMPORARY WORLD ISSUES
Series

Books in the **Contemporary World Issues** series address vital issues in today's society such as genetic engineering, pollution, and biodiversity. Written by professional writers, scholars, and nonacademic experts, these books are authoritative, clearly written, up to date, and objective. They provide a good starting point for research by high school and college students, scholars, and general readers as well as by legislators, businesspeople, activists, and others.

Each book, carefully organized and easy to use, contains an overview of the subject, a detailed chronology, biographical sketches, facts and data and/or documents and other primary source material, a forum of authoritative perspective essays, annotated lists of print and nonprint resources, and an index.

Readers of books in the Contemporary World Issues series will find the information they need in order to have a better understanding of the social, political, environmental, and economic issues facing the world today.

Obesity

A REFERENCE HANDBOOK

SECOND EDITION

Judith S. Stern and Alexandra Kazaks

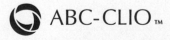

ABC-CLIO™

An Imprint of ABC-CLIO, LLC
Santa Barbara, California • Denver, Colorado

Library of Congress Cataloging-in-Publication Data

Stern, Judith S., 1943– , author.
  Obesity : a reference handbook / Judith S. Stern and Alexandra Kazaks. — Second edition.
      p. ; cm. — (Contemporary world issues)
  Includes bibliographical references and index.
  ISBN 978-1-4408-3804-0 (alk. paper) —
ISBN 978-1-4408-3805-7 (ebook)
  I. Kazaks, Alexandra, author.   II. Title.   III. Series:
Contemporary world issues.
  [DNLM: 1. Obesity—United States—Handbooks. WD 101]
  RA645.O23 2015
  616.3'98—dc23   2015024913

ISBN: 978-1-4408-3804-0
EISBN: 978-1-4408-3805-7

19 18 17 16 15   1 2 3 4 5

This book is also available on the World Wide Web as an eBook.
Visit www.abc-clio.com for details.

ABC-CLIO
An Imprint of ABC-CLIO, LLC

ABC-CLIO, LLC
130 Cremona Drive, P.O. Box 1911
Santa Barbara, California 93116-1911

This book is printed on acid-free paper ∞

Manufactured in the United States of America

Contents

Preface

Obesity impacts the lives of pregnant women, the unborn, newborn, children, adults, the elderly, and even our pets. But the problem of obesity is not confined to the United States. It is worldwide. In the year 2000, the estimated number of overweight people worldwide exceeded the number of people suffering from malnutrition. And this is not a recent phenomenon—it goes back more than 10,000 years.

Today, in the United States, obesity is not a disease of the rich. People with low incomes tend to be more obese than people with high incomes. This is confounded by the observation that if you are obese, you are more likely to be socially down mobile.

And, obese people are discriminated against and made fun of. Even the medical community discriminates against obese patients. For example, very obese people need bigger beds. The causes of obesity are also simplified—if you didn't eat so much you wouldn't be fat. The cure for obesity is also simplified—just eat less and exercise more. But, in truth, research has shown that food restriction is more important for *weight loss* and exercise is more important to *maintain the weight loss*. If you suddenly stop exercising, you will start to regain the weight. How much exercise is recommended for you to lose more than 5 percent body weight and to keep it off? According to the National Heart, Lung, and Blood Institute of the National Institutes of Health (NIH), one may need to be moderately active (like walking briskly) for more than 300 minutes per week.

Could some of this be due to genetics? For example, we study certain rats and mice whose obesity is clearly due to genetics. In people, this is best seen in identical twins whose body weights are more similar in comparison to fraternal twins.

Clearly, the amount that we eat influences weight gain, weight loss, weight maintenance, and weight regain. In this area, time has not been kind. In the United States, over the last 20 years, portion size has increased. There has been "portion distortion." For example, according to NIH, 20 years ago a bagel was 3 inches in diameter and 140 calories. Today, it is 6 inches in diameter and 350 calories. There is portion distortion in other categories: sodas (6.5 ounces or 82 calories to 20 ounces or 250 calories). To be accurate, the number of portions listed on a 20 ounce bottle of soda is 2.5. But, have you ever seen someone share it with 1.5 other people? Even the size of a blueberry muffin has increased from 1.5 ounces (210 calories) to 5 ounces (500 calories). That's easier to share. But, if you have a bigger portion of food, you eat more even if you do not eat it all.

Obesity: A Reference Handbook will open your eyes to the complex causes of obesity, the use of imprecise definitions, the variety of measures of obesity, and the variety of treatments from diet to behavior to drugs to surgery. For example, obesity can be categorized using a measure called Body Mass Index which is weight (kg)/height^2 (meters). Using BMI, underweight is less than 18.5, normal weight is 18.50–24.99, overweight is 25.0–29.9, and obesity is a BMI > 30. Obesity is then classified into three categories: Obesity 1 (BMI 30–34.9), Obesity 2 (BMI > 35.0–39.9), and Obesity 3 (BMI > 40). Body fat distribution (upper body obesity) also can increase your risk for certain chronic diseases (cancer, coronary vascular disease, and hypertension). Risk is increased in men with a waist circumference of more than 40 inches and in women with a waist circumferences of more than35 inches. When you visualize upper body obesity, think of a "pot belly." If a person has lower body obesity, think about "fat" buttocks and thighs.

If we are not very successful in curing obesity, one solution could be to prevent obesity. Simple, straightforward solutions have been proposed. We could label all manufactured food. But labels are complicated. It's hard to find the information for calories and portion size without a magnifying glass. Another proposal is to change government-funded programs like the school lunch program to provide healthier food.

Our bottom line is that we do not know how to prevent obesity. We need more long-term research. And, we need a lot more funding for obesity research. This will take many years. But this should not be used as an excuse to do nothing until we have the research data. To paraphrase our colleague Dr. David Kritchevsky, "We are making progress with obesity research and the scientific findings are changing over time. But we can't wait to treat the obese because by the time all the evidence is in our patients will be dead."

Obesity

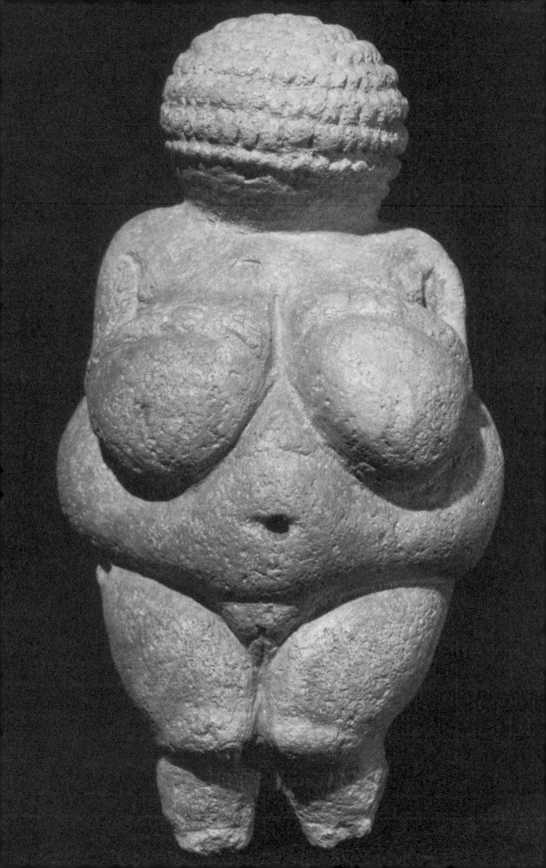

Introduction

Obesity is not a recent phenomenon. Its origins can be traced back to our prehistoric ancestors. Statues dating from the Stone Age provide the earliest depiction of obesity. The Venus of Willendorf, a figurine of an obese woman that dates back to about 22,000 BCE, is thought to represent a fertility goddess. Through the centuries, obesity has been depicted in the arts, literature, and medical opinion both as a highly desirable state and as an unhealthy condition to be avoided. Egyptian temples prominently displayed statues of obese men and women, while medical opinions written on papyrus at the time describe obesity as a disease state. Hippocrates, known as the father of medicine, noted that fat people were more prone to sudden death than were lean people. Stories and chronicles from the Middle Ages portray obese individuals who are wealthy and powerful. Peter Paul Rubens, a well-respected artist of the 17th century, painted ample, robust women who today would be labeled as obese but were considered ideals of female beauty at that time. In 1737, Benjamin Franklin observed in his *Poor Richard's Almanack*: "To lengthen thy life, lessen thy meals" (Franklin 1737). In the 1930s, it was rumored that the Duchess

---

The Venus of Willendorf is a figurine of an obese woman that was unearthed from a Paleolithic archeological site at Willendorf, Austria, in 1908. The image was carved some 25,000 years ago. The statue is about four-and-a-half inches high and has an enlarged stomach and breasts. This body type likely symbolized procreativity, as she was thought to be a fertility goddess. (Ali Meyer/Corbis)

of Windsor declared, "You can never be too rich or too thin," setting a benchmark for socialites then and now.

Although overweight was sometimes linked with disease and a shorter life span, in general, extra fat was related to wealth, health, and attractiveness. Low weight and thinness were associated with poverty, malnutrition, and wasting diseases, such as tuberculosis. Scarcity of food throughout most of history meant that most people did not have the opportunity to become obese. The tendency to store energy in the form of fat results from thousands of years of evolution in an environment characterized by limited or uncertain food supplies. Those who could store energy in times of plenty were more likely to survive periods of famine and to pass this tendency to their offspring. The idea of obesity as a disease with pathologic consequences for a large percentage of the general public is less than a century old. The current availability of inexpensive, high-energy food and the reduced need to expend energy for daily living and work has allowed obesity to become an "equal opportunity" state of health.

Attitudes about body weight have fluctuated with the times. In the mid-19th century, health reformer Sylvester Graham declared that overeating, or gluttony, was a great threat to both health and morality in the United States. In Graham's view, gluttony led to a state of what he called "overstimulation" that would eventually lead to illness and moral failings (Luciano 2001). During America's Gilded Age (1878–1889), fat bodies were equated with fat wallets, while thinness was associated with poverty. Rich men were depicted in the media with gold watch chains stretched across their ample bellies. The fashion of overindulgence was embodied by Diamond Jim Brady, a railroad equipment salesman who was known for his voracious appetite. A typical meal for Brady could include three dozen oysters, six crabs, soup, a half-dozen lobsters, two ducks, steak, vegetables, and a platter of desserts, followed by a two-pound box of candy. When he died at age 56, an autopsy showed his stomach was six times the size of that of a normal man. The fat person as a positive model did not persist past the 19th century.

President William Taft, who weighed 355 pounds when he took office and allegedly suffered the indignity of getting stuck in the White House bathtub, was the last obese president (Luciano 2001).

A number of reasons explain this turnaround in attitudes about fatness. In the early 1920s, movies began to play a major role in shaping ideals of bodily perfection. Movie stars radiated youth, good health, and sex appeal. To look beautiful on film, actors and actresses had to be slim because filming on camera created the illusion that they carried extra pounds. From 1930 into the 1950s, it became fashionable for women to have a fuller bust and slender waist. Women wore girdles to narrow their waists and padded bras to enhance their breast line. Following World War II, fuller shapes became the accepted norm for housewives and mothers. Actresses like Jayne Mansfield and Marilyn Monroe, with their hourglass figures, were the voluptuous female ideal. During the late 1960s and early 1970s, the feminist movement questioned existing female stereotypes. The self-health movement at the time encouraged women to take pride in their bodies. This new concern of women about health and fitness fostered an industry that promoted cellulite creams, exercises to develop so-called buns of steel, and liposuction to remove unwanted fat. After the 1970s, a new, more athletic look became popular as increasing numbers of men and women began to participate in sports and regular exercise. In spite of the continuing popularity of the athletic body type, the prevailing look among top fashion models has remained ultrathin.

Through television, movies, and magazines, the media set unrealistic standards for desirable body weight and appearance. And portrayal of what is attractive and healthy keeps getting thinner and thinner for women and more muscular for men. At the beginning of the 21st century, two-thirds of Americans were overweight. In the coming decades, the population is expected to include a greater proportion of older people. The media image of health and beauty will be increasingly out of step with a population that is growing older and fatter.

The belief that weight and health could—and should—be under one's personal control generated a proliferation of dieting plans and treatments. One of the first commercially available diets came from William Banting in 1864. It was based on a high-protein and high-fat "low farinaceous" plan recommended to him by his doctor. Enthusiastic about his weight loss, he published the diet as "A Letter on Corpulence, Addressed to the Public" (Banting 1865). The plan became so popular that people spoke of "banting" when they went on any weight loss diet. Before the pure food and drug laws were passed in the United States, individuals seeking a cure-all for obesity were treated with doses of such products as vinegar and soap. Other ingredients used extensively in the 1920s that produced almost instant weight reduction were laxatives, which cause diarrhea, and purgatives, which induce vomiting. In the early 1900s, popular weight loss drugs included a wide array of animal-derived thyroid extracts, arsenic, and strychnine. Each could cause temporary weight loss, but they were unsafe to use. Newspapers of the time carried advertisements for Kellogg's Safe Fat Reducer, a much-promoted remedy that contained an extract of animal thyroid glands. Through a combination of aggressive advertising and questionable ethics, Kellogg's became a popular remedy for people seeking rapid weight loss. It was eventually revealed that the Safe Fat Reducer was a combination of thyroid extract, some laxatives, and breadcrumbs. Thyroid hormone, as the active ingredient, increased risk of hypertension, cardiac arrest, and stroke. Long-term use could result in loss of normal thyroid function, osteoporosis, increased heart rate, sweating, chest pain, and sudden death. The American Medical Association was successful in getting the thyroid extract removed from the product. However, it remained on the market and sold simply as a laxative.

For decades, thyroid hormone was medically prescribed for obesity with the hope that an increase in metabolic rate would result in weight loss. Long-term studies demonstrated that weight loss occurring during thyroid hormone administration was due in part to the breakdown of vital protein as well as unwanted fat. In the 1930s, doctors prescribed dinitrophenol, a benzene-derived ingredient in World War I explosives. Dinitrophenol did increase metabolism and produced weight loss, but the drug was abandoned because of severe side effects, including neuropathy and cataracts. During that time, it was legal to sell untested remedies because drug makers were not required to prove that their products were safe before they were put on the market.

Defining and Measuring Overweight and Obesity

Defining overweight and obesity is somewhat subjective and imprecise. "Overweight" is defined as having more body weight than is considered normal or healthy for one's age or build. The term "obese" is used for very overweight people who have a high percentage of body fat. Normal weights have been variously referred to as "ideal," "desirable," or "healthy." In addition to these subjective terms are several objective measures that are used to classify individual weight.

Indirect Measuring Methods
Height-Weight Tables
In 1942, Louis Dublin, a statistician at Metropolitan Life Insurance Company, grouped some 4 million people who were insured with Metropolitan Life into categories based on their height, body frame (small, medium, or large), and weight. He discovered that those who lived the longest were the people who maintained their body weight at a level that was average for 25-year-olds. The results were published in the Metropolitan Life standard height-weight tables for men and women. This statistical analysis of national averages of weight relative to age, sex, and height became the accepted recommendations for a healthy

weight (Greville 1947). The "1942–1943 Metropolitan Height and Weight Tables" (see Tables 5.1 and 5.2) were widely used for determining "ideal" body weights.

In 1959, research indicated that the lowest mortality rates were associated with lower-than-average weights, and the phrase "desirable weight" replaced "ideal weight" in the height and weight table (MLIC 1959). The weights were derived from those weight-for-height proportions associated with lowest mortality among people in the United States and Canada who purchased life insurance policies from 1935 to 1954. However, these weights were associated with the lowest death rates but not necessarily with the lowest morbidity (rate of illness or disease). In 1983, the tables were revised once again and called simply "height and weight tables." The weights given in the 1983 tables are heavier than the 1942 tables because, in general, heavier people were living longer (MLIC 1983). It is interesting to note that neither medical nor academic experts were the authoritative voices in setting weight guidelines. It was the life insurance industry that established the system of weight classification that became part of medical practice throughout the United States.

A number of criticisms surrounded the use of a table to determine whether an individual is at the right weight—or even what "ideal weight" means. Experts have criticized the validity of the Metropolitan Life tables for several reasons:

- Insured people tend to be healthier than uninsured people.
- Frame size was not consistently measured.
- The tables were based on a predominantly white, middle-class population.
- Some individuals were actually weighed and some reported their estimated weight.
- Height and weight were measured in people wearing shoes and clothing of varying amounts and weights.

- Both smokers and nonsmokers were included. Smoking is a significant factor that increases risk of disease and death.

Thus, height-weight tables provided only a general health guide, and other measurements should be included for overall evaluation of well-being.

People in the United States were able to find out how much they weighed when penny scales were imported from Germany in the 1880s. Soon after, the National Scale Company manufactured the first coin-operated scales in the United States. These scales were among the first automatic vending machines. Being able to weigh oneself was a novelty at the time, and during the 1920s and 1930s, coin-operated scales appeared in drugstores in almost every city and town. In the 1940s, improvements in mechanical scale technology made inexpensive personal scales available for in-home use. Today, we can choose bathroom scales that are digital, or that are solar powered, or that "talk" and say the weight aloud. The accuracy in these scales may vary, but they serve the general purpose of measuring whether body weight is going up or down.

Estimated Ideal Body Weight

In 1964, Dr. G. J. Hamwi developed a simple rule for estimating ideal body weight (IBW). The Hamwi formulas became very popular when they first appeared in a publication of the American Diabetes Association (Hamwi 1964). They have remained a well-accepted method of calculating ideal weight in clinical situations. The formulas for IBW are:

- Men—106 pounds for the first 5 feet; 6 pounds for each inch over 5 feet
- Women—100 pounds for the first 5 feet; 5 pounds for each inch over 5 feet

In addition, a range of 10 percent variation above or below the calculated weight was allowed for individual differences.

Example:

The estimated IBW of a man who is 5 feet 11 inches tall would be calculated as: 106 + (6 × 11) = 106 + 66 = 172 pounds

The range with 10 percent variation below and above is 155–189 pounds (10% of 172 = about 17 pounds, so 172 – 17 = 155 and 172 + 17 = 189).

The estimated IBW of a woman who is 5 feet 4 inches tall would be calculated as: 100 + (5 × 4) = 100 + 20 = 120 pounds

The range with 10 percent variation below and above is 113–137 pounds (10% of 120 = 12 pounds, so 125 – 12 = 113 and 125 + 12 = 137).

The IBW does not correlate weight to health or prevention of disease. One criticism of the IBW formula is that it does not allow for body composition or body type. Someone with large bones or with a high percentage of lean tissue (muscle) would appear to be overweight, according to this method. For some, the IBW may be an unrealistic range, and they may try unnecessary or fad dieting to reach the "ideal" number.

Body Mass Index

As definitions of overweight have varied widely, health experts have struggled to develop a useful definition of healthy weight. Their recommendations have evolved from weight-for-height standards to sex-specific references. The most recent proposal is to use a single number, the body mass index (BMI) that is applied to all adults. BMI is a calculated number, based on height and weight of an individual. It is calculated as:

BMI = weight (lb)/[height (in)] 2 × 703 (standard units of measure)

or

BMI = weight (kg)/[height (m)] 2 (metric units of measure)
where kg = kilogram, m = meter, lb = pound, and in = inch.

This number is used to assess the relationship of body weight to health and disease risk. Because it is independent of age and reference population, BMI can be used for comparisons across studies both in the United States and internationally. The BMI is more generous than the IBW. BMI calculations are meant to be applied only to adults over the age of 20.

BMI can be calculated in inches and pounds (in the United States) or in meters and kilograms (in countries that use the metric system).

One can calculate BMI by dividing weight in pounds by height in inches squared and multiplying that number by a conversion factor of 703.

Example:

If one's weight is 150 pounds and height is 5 feet 5 inches tall (65 inches), the BMI is calculated as: [150 ÷ (65)2] × 703 = 24.96

With the metric system, the formula for BMI is weight in kilograms divided by height in meters squared.

Example:

If one's weight is 68 kilograms and height is 165 centimeters (1.65 meters), the BMI is calculated as: 68 ÷ (1.65)2 = 24.98

One can use available tables to easily determine BMI (see Table 5.3) or enter one's weight and height into a Web-based BMI calculator. One such calculator is available on the Centers for Disease Control and Prevention (CDC) "Body Mass Index" page at http://www.cdc.gov/nccdphp/dnpa/bmi/

Based on guidelines from the National Heart, Lung and Blood Institute and the World Health Organization, Table 1.1 shows weight ranges compared with BMI values used to determine weight status.

The BMI was first developed in the mid-1800s by Belgian mathematician Adolphe Quetelet. Quetelet worked with life insurance companies to determine factors related to birth and death. These types of correlations using body weight are common now, but in 1833 the idea was revolutionary. More recently, governmental agencies and scientific health organizations have defined a BMI that correlates with possible health risks of overweight by using a statistically derived definition from a series of cross-sectional surveys called the National Health and Nutrition Examination Surveys (NHANES). These surveys are designed to gather information on the health and nutritional status of the population of the United States. From 1985 to 1998, the definition of overweight in government publications was a BMI of at least 27.3 for women and 27.8 for men.

Table 1.1   Weight Ranges, BMI Values, and Weight Status

Height	Weight Range	BMI	Considered
5 feet 9 inches	124 lb. or less	Below 18.5	Underweight
	125 lb. to 168 lb.	18.5–24.9	Healthy weight
	169 lb. to 202 lb.	25.0–29.9	Overweight
	203 lb. or more	30 or higher	Obese

Note: This example is specific for a person 5 feet 9 inches tall.

Source: CDC (2007a).

In 1995, the World Health Organization recommended a new classification system that included three "grades" of overweight using BMI cutoff points of 25, 30, and 40. The International Obesity Task Force suggested an additional cutoff point of 35. Eventually, in June 1998, an expert panel convened by the National Institutes of Health (NIH) released a report that identified being overweight as having a BMI between 25 and 29.9 and being obese as having a BMI of 30 or above. These definitions, widely used by the federal government and increasingly used by the broader medical and scientific communities, are based on evidence that health risks increase more steeply in individuals with a BMI greater than 25. The term "morbid obesity" is still used for medical coding purposes for individuals with a BMI of 40 or above; however, the NIH recommends the use of other descriptive terms, such as "Class III obesity," "extreme obesity," or "clinically severe obesity."

Use of BMI cutoffs has been varied, yielding contrasting results. A shift in BMI criteria can have a large effect on the population at risk (Kuczmarski and Flegal 2000). For example, when applying the BMI cutoffs of ≥27.8 for men and ≥27.3 for women to NHANES III—data collected between 1988 and 1994—the prevalence of overweight is 33 percent for men and 36 percent for women (CDC 1999). In contrast, with the lower BMI cutoff of ≥25.0, the prevalence is 59 percent among men and 51 percent among women. Changing the overweight group cutoff increases the estimated number of overweight adults from 61.7 million to 97.1 million, putting 35.4 million more adults into the overweight category.

Limitations and Shortcomings: Measuring body weight and body dimensions—or anthropometry—is a quick and inexpensive way to estimate body fatness. However, using calculated numbers, such as the BMI, does have limitations. A problem with using BMI as a measurement tool is that very muscular people may be classified as overweight when they are actually healthy. Similarly, people who have lost muscle mass, such as elderly individuals, may have a body weight that seems to be in the healthy BMI category when they actually have a high percentage of body fat. The health risks associated with overweight and obesity are based on a continuum and do not necessarily correspond to strict cutoff points. For example, an overweight individual with a BMI of 29 does not substantially add to his or her health consequences simply by moving up one notch to a BMI of 30, the threshold of the obese category (WIN 2006). Because health risks generally do increase with increasing BMI, it is a useful screening tool for individuals and a general guideline to monitor trends in the population. By itself, BMI is not diagnostic for individual health status. Further assessment should be performed to evaluate associated health risks.

BMI ranges for children and teens (aged 2–19 years old) are defined so that they take into account normal differences between boys and girls at various ages. After BMI is calculated, the BMI number is plotted on BMI-for-age growth charts specific for either girls or boys to obtain a percentile ranking. The percentile indicates the relative position of the child's BMI number among children of the same sex and age. The Centers for Disease Control and Prevention BMI-for-age weight status categories and the corresponding percentiles are shown in Table 1.2.

The CDC provides more information about BMI for children and teens on an interactive Web site, "About BMI for Children and Teens," at http://www.cdc.gov/nccdphp/dnpa/

Table 1.2   Children's BMI-for-Age Weight Status

Weight Status Category	Percentile Range (compared with boys or girls of same age)
Underweight	Less than the 5th percentile
Healthy weight	5th percentile to less than the 85th percentile
At risk of overweight	85th to less than the 95th percentile
Overweight	Equal to or greater than the 95th percentile

Source: CDC (2007a).

healthyweight/assessing/bmi/childrens_BMI/about_child
rens_BMI.htm

Debate is ongoing among researchers and health professionals about whether BMI is a reasonable indicator of body fatness, as the correlation between the BMI and body fatness can
vary greatly according to sex, age, and race. For example:

- At the same BMI, women tend to have more body fat
  than men.
- At the same BMI, older people, on average, tend to have
  more body fat than younger adults.
- Race and ethnicity issues are inherent in BMI measurements.

BMI does not take into account how people of different races
and ethnicities vary in muscle mass versus fat mass. People of
African and Polynesian ancestry may have less body fat and
more lean muscle mass for a given weight, and thus a higher
baseline BMI for overweight and obesity may be appropriate
for these populations. At the other end of the scale, one study
found that current BMI thresholds significantly underestimate
health risks in many non-Europeans (Gallagher 2004). The
body fat percentage of an Asian may be higher than that of a
Caucasian of the same height and weight. Even within normal
BMI ranges, Asian groups can have a high risk of weight-related
health problems, and they could begin to have abnormalities in
their blood glucose levels above a BMI of just 21. It has been
suggested that BMI levels be dropped to 23 and 25 to indicate
overweight and obesity, respectively, among Asian populations
(Razak et al. 2007).

Assessing Percentage of Body Fat

BMI is not a specific index of fatness because its numerator—
measured body weight—may reflect muscle, bone, or body
water in addition to fat. The percentage of body fat is difficult
to measure directly. Fat, or adipose, tissue is stored underneath

the skin as subcutaneous fat; as intramuscular fat, interspersed in skeletal muscle; and as visceral adipose tissue, found deep in the body around vital organs. Body fat can be divided into two categories according to its physiological purpose: Essential fat cushions and insulates organs and is necessary for normal body function. Nonessential fat is excess energy stored away for future use. Although no universal body fat standards are in place, the American Council on Exercise has suggested an average amount of body fat of 18–24 percent for men and 25–31 percent for women. Any amount over that range would be considered obesity (ACSM 2001).

The distribution of adipose tissue is important, because overweight and obese adults are assigned to risk categories depending on body shape and location of fat deposits. "Pear-shaped" individuals, who have fat deposits on their hips and thighs, are less susceptible to obesity-related diseases than "apple-shaped" people, who store fat in the abdominal area. Abdominal fat accumulation is generally considered to be a key health risk indicator, as increased waist circumference is associated strongly with cardiovascular disease and is a good predictor of future risk of type 2 diabetes and all-cause mortality. Measuring waist circumference is a simple procedure that provides information about fat distribution, but it is unclear how commonly clinicians measure waist circumference. Anecdotal evidence suggests that this practice is not routine. As part of a complete health risk assessment, health care professionals are urged to incorporate waist circumference along with measuring weight, height, and BMI calculations (Ford, Mokdad, and Giles 2003).

Direct Measuring Methods: Direct measures of body fat include underwater weighing, bioelectrical impedance analysis (BIA), dual energy X-ray absorptiometry (DEXA), and skinfold thickness. These measures of body fat can be expensive or time consuming, and are not normally used by primary care clinicians. However, they can complement BMI to assess risk and monitor the progress of therapeutic interventions (Erselcan et al. 2000).

Underwater Weighing: Underwater weighing, also known as densitometry or hydrostatic weighing, has long been the gold standard for determining body composition (relative amounts of fat and lean). This technique involves weighing a person when dry, and then measuring his or her weight when totally submerged in a tub of water and the air in the lungs has been fully exhaled. It is based on Archimedes' principle, which states that given an equal weight, lower-density objects have a larger surface area and displace more water than higher-density objects. Bone and muscle are denser than water and sinks, and fat is less dense than water and floats. Of two individuals of the same weight but with different proportions of fat and lean, the one with the most body fat weighs less underwater. The volume of water displaced by a person and the difference between the dry weight and the submerged weight are entered into equations that can be used to estimate the percentage of body fat. The primary disadvantages of this method are the cost and time required, the subject having to be underwater, and the variability in the ability of individuals to fully exhale. This technique is not a useful approach for large-scale studies, and in terms of precision, a DEXA scan is an alternative.

Dual Energy X-Ray Absorptiometry: With DEXA, a scanner measures body composition using low-energy X-rays. This method was originally developed to not only evaluate changes in bone mineral density, but it also reveals total body composition. DEXA works by passing two X-ray beams through the individual and measuring the amount of X-ray absorbed by the tissue it has passed through. One beam is high intensity and one is low intensity, so the relative absorbance of each beam is an indication of the density of the tissue. DEXA differentiates fat from lean mass, as the tissue with greater density (e.g., bone and muscle) shows a greater reduction in X-ray that passes through and that can be detected. The amount of radiation energy that is used with DEXA is extremely small. It would take approximately 800 full-body DEXA scans to equal the exposure to the amount of radiation received from one standard chest X-ray. The level of radiation is low enough that DEXA is approved by the U.S. Food and Drug Administration as a screening device to predict body composition. DEXA is a very accurate measure of body fat, although it is expensive and is generally limited to clinical research studies (Bolanowski and Nilsson 2001).

Bioelectrical Impedance Analysis: BIA is based on the principle that body tissue is capable of conducting electricity. Water is a good conductor of electricity, and most body water is found in lean tissue. Fat, which has almost no water in it, is such a poor conductor of electricity that it actually impedes, or slows down, the electrical flow. High measured resistance equals a high level of fat. Impedance is calculated by entering the resistance data into regression equations that take into account the person's weight, age, gender, and ethnicity. The BIA method is population specific, and an equation must be used that is specific to the population being measured (Heymsfield et al. 1996). Although this type of measurement initially required a laboratory procedure that involved attaching electrodes to the hands and feet, the technology now features easy-to-use devices, including at-home floor scales. BIA is considered to be safe because BIA currents (at a frequency of 50 kHz) are unlikely to stimulate electrically excitable tissues, such as nerves or cardiac muscle. The small current magnitudes are less than the threshold of perception—that is, they are not noticeable. Anyone with an implanted defibrillator should avoid BIA evaluation because even small currents could potentially provoke an incorrect defibrillator response (NHLBI 1998).

Skinfold Measurement: Skinfold measurement is an inexpensive option for estimating body fat based on the assumption that subcutaneous fat reflects the total fat content of the body. Calipers are used to measure subcutaneous fat at specific sites around the body, including chest, hip, abdomen, thigh, and upper arm. Prediction equations that help estimate body fat from skinfold sites can be examined in Table 5.4.

The skinfold technique is prone to significant measurement errors. Limitations on how wide the calipers open can make skinfold measurement challenging to use with extremely obese patients. In addition, not all body fat, such as intra-abdominal and intramuscular fat, is accessible to the calipers, and the distribution of subcutaneous fat can vary significantly throughout the human body. Although skinfold measurements are easily administered and are practical for large studies, they have been found to provide the least accurate estimates of percentage of body fat (Wang et al. 2000).

Obesity Trends in the United States

In 1985, the CDC began releasing maps examining the changes in U.S. average BMI over time and the variation in BMI among the states. Though not all states participated in the CDC survey, none of those that reported had an obesity rate above 15 percent. Obesity looks like an epidemic that is initiated in states in the Southeast, but continued to increase in all states. Obesity prevalence in states with the highest rates got higher and higher over time. To maintain validity, the methods to collect national data were adapted to the changing modes of communication in that year. However, it means that estimates from data collected in 2010 and before cannot be directly compared to estimates from data collected in 2011 and forward (CDC 2014a).

In 2014, an estimated two-thirds (67%) of U.S. adults could be classified as either overweight or obese. Of those, about 34 percent were in the obese category (Ogden, 2014). It means that there were as many Americans who were obese as those who were just overweight. Since the 1980s, obesity rates for adults have doubled and rates for children have tripled. Prevalence of obesity has increased among all groups regardless of age, sex, ethnicity, socioeconomic status, or geographic region. In 2013, obesity was most common in Mississippi and West Virginia where at least 35 percent of adults were obese, and rarest in Colorado, with about 21 percent obesity (CDC 2014a).

A growing body of evidence suggests that obesity is considerably influenced by social variables such as gender roles and ethnicity. The prevalence of obesity is increasing among all age and

racial groups in the United States. There is, however, a disproportionate rise in the prevalence of obesity among blacks (African Americans) and Mexican Americans, especially in women,
when compared to whites in the United States. Non-Hispanic
blacks have the highest age-adjusted rates of obesity (47.8%),
followed by Hispanics (42.5%), non-Hispanic whites (32.6%),
and non-Hispanic Asians (10.8%) (CDC 2014a).

Statistics not shown in these maps, but of even greater concern, are that there were 30 states in which the percentage of
obese or overweight children was 30 percent or more. Childhood obesity prevalence has not changed significantly since
2003 and remains at about 17 percent (Ogden 2014). A young
person with excess weight has a high risk of obesity-related
health problems in the future. Overweight adolescents have
a 70 percent chance of becoming overweight or obese adults.
Heart disease related to high cholesterol and high blood pressure occurs with increased frequency in overweight young
people compared with those with a healthy weight. Type 2
diabetes, closely linked to overweight and obesity and previously considered an adult disease, has increased significantly
in children and adolescents. Experts had serious concerns that
the current generation of children would experience debilitating chronic diseases in adulthood and would actually have a
shorter life span than their parents (Olshansky 2005).

However, after decades of increases in national obesity, a
2010 analysis of NHANES data suggested that increases in
overweight and obesity had slowed or perhaps had reached a
plateau. Compared with the previous 10-year period, the analysis showed:

- 32.2 percent of men were obese compared with 27 percent
  in 1999. However, there had been no significant change in
  obesity rates since 2003.
- 35.5 percent of women were obese compared with 33.4 percent in 1999. The increase was not statistically significant.

- 31.7 percent of children were obese or overweight compared with 29 percent in 1999. This increase also was not a statistically significant difference (Flegal 2010).

Even though these findings were good news, most Americans are still overweight and one-third is obese. Epidemiologists with the CDC's National Center for Health Statistics report that, though the obesity trend appears to be slowing down, the prevalence remains unacceptably high, and obesity continues to be a serious national health concern (CDC 2010).

The most rapidly increasing trend in obesity has occurred in the obese adult population who has extreme or severe obesity (a BMI of 40 or greater and more than 100 pounds of extra weight). In a study of extreme weight category trends between the years 1986 and 2000, the prevalence of a BMI of 40 or greater quadrupled from about one in 200 adult Americans to one in 50. The prevalence of a BMI of 50 went from about one individual in 2000 to one in 400. This increase included males and females, all ethnic groups, all age groups, and all education levels. Those with the highest BMI at the baseline measurement had the greatest increases.

Obesity as a National Health Problem

When Brandreth Symonds, a life insurance statistician, published "The Influence of Overweight and Underweight on Vitality" in 1908, his statistical analysis of insurance policyholders showed that overweight was a greater risk factor for a shortened life span than underweight. Dr. Symonds wrote, "Speaking generally, it is safer to be thin than fat" (Symonds 1908).

In 1943, enough of the U.S. population was above the IBW, so much so that the Metropolitan Life Insurance Company declared, "Overweight is so common that it constitutes a national health problem of the first order" (MLIC 1943). In a classic paper, Dr. Lester Breslow noted that "one out of six 'well people'. . . were 20 percent or more overweight" and that weight control was a "major public health problem" (Breslow 1952). The obesity prevalence estimates in Breslow's paper are small compared with the current figures showing that 65 percent of U.S. adults are now classified as overweight or obese. Former U.S. Surgeon General David Satcher declared obesity to be a "public health epidemic" in the 2001 publication "Surgeon General's Call to Action to Prevent and Decrease Overweight and Obesity." He said, "Health problems resulting from overweight and obesity could reverse many of the health gains achieved in the U.S. in recent decades" (USDHHS 2001).

Healthy People 2010, a U.S. Department of Health and Human Services health promotion and disease prevention program, highlighted overweight and obesity as key indicators of national health. It set an objective to reduce the prevalence of obesity among adults to less than 15 percent. Current data indicate that the obesity situation is getting worse, and unfortunately, no progress was made toward the Healthy People 2010 target of 15 percent reduction in obesity in the United States. Instead, prevalence of obesity increased 47.8 percent. The proportion of adults in the population who were obese rose from 23 to 34 percent. During the same period, obesity increased in children from 11 to 17 percent and in adolescents from 11 to 18 percent moving away from the 2010 targets of just 5 percent (CDC, 2013). Current goals for Healthy People 2020 are just to "reduce the proportion" of adults, children, and adolescents who are considered obese (USDHHS, 2014).

Why Are We Overweight?

The obesity crisis did not happen overnight. It has been developing for decades, but only recently has it attracted much public attention. The U.S. population has experienced steady gains in both weight and height since the late 19th century. These gains improved our capability to withstand diseases and increased our longevity. Between 1900 and 2000, life expectancy at birth in the United States increased by 65 percent for women and 60 percent for men. Gains in height among U.S. adults have leveled off, and weight has continued to increase. As obesity and overweight have risen in our population, the greatest increase in the past two decades has been seen in the prevalence of extreme obesity. Those who are severely obese are most at risk for serious health problems (NHLBI 1998; NIH 1998).

Most people are aware of the health problems associated with excess weight. Diet books top the best-seller list and the electronic and print media are loaded with nutrition advice, but successful individual weight management is haphazard or even nonexistent. Why are Americans overweight? Is it the availability of fast food? Oversized portions? Too much TV? Experts argue about the causes or contributors to overweight and obesity, but the realistic answer is, too many calories. The reality is that we eat too much and move too little. At the most fundamental level, weight gain is caused by the imbalance between food and activity: too much energy in and too little energy out. Weight gain is the normal physiologic response that occurs when energy intake exceeds energy expenditure.

Obesity is a consequence of our modern life. We have access to large amounts of palatable, high-calorie food and a limited need for physical activity. Humans evolved in an environment that required vigorous physical activity and was characterized by cyclical feast and famine. To survive, humans developed an innate preference for sweet and fatty foods. These natural defenses against starvation go awry in an environment where food is always plentiful and technology has reduced the need for human physical work. As the amount of energy, or calories, in our food supply has grown in recent decades, each person consumed more food. Those extra calories turn into extra pounds year after year.

Food energy is measured in calories. A calorie is defined as the amount of energy (or heat) it takes to raise 1 gram of water (approximately 1 cubic centimeter, or about a thimbleful) 1°C. In nutrition terms, the word "calorie" is used instead of the more precise scientific term "kilocalorie" or 1,000 calories of energy. Dietary calories are in fact kilocalories (Kcal), with the "kilo-" prefix omitted. Here, the terms are interchangeable, with Kcal used most often with numbers or measurements.

When extra energy in the form of protein (4 Kcal/gram), fat (9 Kcal/gram), carbohydrate (4 Kcal/gram) and/or alcohol (7 Kcal/gram) is consumed, the excess energy is stored in the form of body fat. Conversely, by limiting energy intake, body fat loss will be in proportion to the calorie deficit. Each pound of body fat represents approximately 3,500 Kcal. Reducing calorie intake by 500 Kcal per day theoretically results in a 1 pound per week weight loss. Small changes in food intake can make large differences over time. For example, using one tablespoon of mayonnaise on a sandwich instead of two tablespoons can save 100 calories per day. Over a year, the total 36,500 Kcal (365 days × 100 Kcal/day) deficit could mean a loss of 10 pounds of body fat. Most people have between 25 billion and 35 billion fat cells. This number can increase in response to excessive weight gain to as many as 150 billion cells. Fat cells expand and shrink in size during weight gain and loss, but they never disappear.

Because resting metabolic rate (the energy required to maintain basic physiologic functions and for digestion) varies widely among individuals, calorie intake and physical energy expenditure are the most variable components of energy balance. Changes in eating and activity provide the best opportunities to prevent or treat obesity (Goran 2000).

Despite concern about the increasing levels of obesity, and the knowledge that it is caused by excess energy intake and low levels of physical activity, obesity remains a poorly understood phenomenon. Considerable gaps remain in our knowledge about the physiological pathways underlying weight gain and the effectiveness of dietary, behavioral, and physical activity interventions. Americans, among the heaviest people on Earth, are becoming fatter and at an ever younger age. How we got to this point is an account of the complex interplay between biological, psychosocial, and economic factors.

Factors That Contribute to Obesity

To understand obesity, we must comprehend the dimensions of energy balance:

Energy in: Factors that affect food consumption

Energy out: Factors that affect activity level

Metabolic, genetic, and behavioral contributions

Increased Energy Intake

The surge in obesity in the United States reflects about a 25 percent increase in per capita energy intake between 1970 and 2000. The U.S. Department of Agriculture's (USDA's) Economic Research Service (ERS) data suggest that average daily calorie consumed went from 2,220 Kcal to 2,680 Kcal. These figures are estimated from the total food available in the national supply (Miller 2015). Several factors have encouraged Americans to eat more. In the early 1980s, food production was an average of 3,300 calories a day for every person. Then, the U.S. farm policy changed, in a way that moved farmers toward lower price supports, greater planting flexibility, and greater orientation to market forces. Farmers increased harvests and no longer plowed under food crops to get subsidies for reducing production. Today, American farmers produce enough food to allow every person 3,900 calories a day. Food prices in stores and restaurants have been declining relative to prices of all other items. Between 1952 and 2003, the ratio of food prices to the price of all other goods fell by 12 percent. Foods that once were available only seasonally are now available year-round, and advances in food processing and packaging have made available a multitude of ready-to-eat foods virtually anywhere at any time (Variyam 2005).

"A Nation at Risk: Obesity in the United States," published jointly by the American Heart Association and the Robert Wood Johnson Foundation in 2005, reported data from scientific research studies about changes in the eating patterns of Americans over the past few decades. Trends that contribute to obesity are:

1. More calories: Adults consumed approximately 300 more calories daily in 2000 than they did in 1985.
2. Bigger portion sizes: A study in the *Journal of the American Medical Association*, cited in this study, reported a significant rise in portion sizes from 1977 to 1996.
3. A major increase in eating out: Spending in fast-food restaurants grew 18 times (from $6 billion to $110 billion) in the past three decades. In 1970, approximately 30,000 fast-food restaurants were operating in the United States; in 2001, approximately 222,000 were in operation (AHA 2005).

Distorted Portion Sizes

Portion sizes have dramatically increased in the past 40 years. As we are exposed to larger quantities of food sold as a single portion, we become victims of "portion distortion." Many of the changes have been too subtle to notice; we have become used to larger servings, and we now expect them. Consider the maximum serving size of french fries sold at McDonald's. It has increased from 210 calories in 1955 to 610 calories. Greater increases are seen in the size of soft drinks. In the 1950s, the standard-size Coca Cola was about 6 ounces. At many U.S. convenience stores, 64-ounce (2 quarts) soft drinks are common.

The sizes of muffins, bagels, and croissants also contribute to portion distortion. Portion-size increases have been continuous since the 1970s. In a sample of 63,380 individuals who responded to national surveys conducted by the USDA between

1977 and 1998, food portion sizes consumed at home and in restaurants increased markedly (Nielsen and Popkin 2003):

- Salty snacks increased from 1.0 to 1.6 ounces = 93 more calories.
- Soft drinks increased from 13.1 to 19.9 fluid ounces = 49 more calories.
- Hamburgers increased from 5.7 to 7.0 ounces = 97 more calories.
- Mexican food increased from 6.3 to 8.0 ounces = 133 more calories.

Though it only costs a few cents more to get a larger size of french fries or a soft drink, the result is too many calories for one person. "Value meals" may not generate any savings when the monetary and psychological costs of trying to lose weight gained from eating larger portions are factored in. Large portion sizes are not limited to meals. Bags of snack foods or soft drinks in vending machines and grocery stores are available in larger and larger sizes that contain multiple servings. (The NIH Web site, "Portion Distortion," has an interactive quiz to show how portions today compare with portion sizes 20 years ago. Visit http://hp2010.nhlbihin.net/portion/ to view the quiz.)

What is the effect of larger portion sizes on food intake? According to research conducted by Professor Brian Wansink, people eat more if the product is being eaten from larger packages (Wansink and Kim 2005). He conducted a "popcorn test" demonstrating that people given large containers of popcorn ate an average of 44 percent more (equal to about 120 Kcal) than those who were given small containers, even though they said the popcorn did not taste very good. In a study by Rolls and colleagues, volunteers ate 30 percent more macaroni and cheese when given large 35 ounce portions than when they were given smaller 18 ounce portions during a meal (Rolls,

Morris, and Roe 2002). Consumers eat more from large servings, but, more important, they also get a distorted impression of what a reasonable serving size really is.

Large food portions affect children's energy intake at meals, even among toddlers (Fisher et al. 2007). Children ranging in age from two to nine years were either given an age-appropriate entrée at the dinner meal or a portion size twice as large as the age-appropriate portion. The study results showed that children as young as two years had a 13 percent higher energy intake at the meal when given the large-portion entrée. Interestingly, children took a similar number of bites regardless of the portion size, but they took bigger bites when served the larger portion.

What Is the Difference between Portion Size and Serving Size?

Portion control is not easy. Standardized servings, used to develop labeling laws and the USDA Dietary Guidelines, are much smaller than portions commonly consumed. Portion size is the amount of a single food item served in a single eating occasion, such as a meal or a snack. A portion is the amount offered to a person in a restaurant, the amount offered in the packaging of prepared foods, or the quantity a person chooses to put on his or her plate.

Serving size is a standardized unit of measuring foods—for example, a cup or an ounce—used in the Dietary Guidelines for Americans and listed on a product label's nutrition facts. The portion and serving size may match, but frequently they are different. For example, bagels or muffins are often sold in portion sizes that comprise at least two servings. When consumers eat the whole product, they may think that they have eaten only a single serving (CDC 2006).

Food labels can help people understand that portions are often larger than they think. For example, one serving of potato or corn chips might supply just 100 calories. But when the serving size is only 10 chips and there are 10 servings per bag, the calories really add up if a person finishes the whole bag. The Nutrition Facts Labels on beverage containers often give the calories for only part of the contents. The label on a 20-ounce bottle often lists the number of calories in an 8-ounce serving, even though the bottle contains 20 ounces or 2.5 servings. To figure out how many calories are in the whole bottle, one must multiply the number of calories in one serving by the number of servings in the bottle (100 × 2.5). The whole bottle actually contains 250 calories. It is important to look closely at the serving size when determining the calorie content of beverages. Note that the serving size on the Nutrition Facts Label is not a recommended amount of food to eat; it is just the calories and nutrients in a given amount of food.

Drinking More Calories

Sugar-sweetened beverages, including sweetened fruit drinks and carbonated drinks, account for nearly half of the added sugars in the U.S. diet (Guthrie and Morton 2000). In 1997, 2.8 million vending machines dispensed more than 27 billion drinks. Most of those drinks came in 12-ounce cans, but the soft drink trend is toward serving sizes of 20 ounces or more. The larger the container, the more beverage people will drink, especially when they assume that the container is a single serving, whether it is 12 ounces, 20 ounces, or more (Johnson et al. 2007). Soft drinks contribute extra energy that adds up day after day, and eventually leads to overweight and obesity. During 2009–2010, U.S. adults consumed an estimated average of 151 kcal per day of sweetened beverages (MMWR 2014).

Another reason to limit sugar-sweetened drinks is that liquid calories may not be recognized by the body's appetite feedback mechanisms. People normally adjust or moderate energy intake by eating less after a large meal, but that moderation occurs more readily with solid foods than with beverages. This phenomenon was seen in a study of men and women who were given 450 extra calories per day as either 3–12-ounce cans of soda or 45 large jelly beans. The people who ate the candy adjusted for the extra energy and later ate less. Those who got the extra liquid calories made no compensation afterward; subsequently, their overall calorie intake increased. The author of the article stated, "Liquid calories don't trip our satiety mechanisms. They just don't register" (DiMeglio and Mattes 2000).

Conveniently Available Food

Some of the observed increase in caloric intake may be associated with the increase in eating out. Data from USDA's food intake surveys show that the food away-from-home sector provided 32 percent of total food energy consumption in 1994–1996, up from 18 percent in 1977–1978. The data also suggest that, when eating out, people either eat more or eat higher calorie foods—or both—and that this tendency appears to be increasing.

Meals eaten away from home allow easy and often inexpensive access to large quantities of calorie-rich foods. In 1970, away-from-home meals represented 25 percent of households' total food budget. That share rose to its highest level of 43.1 percent by 2012. A number of factors contributed to the trend of increased dining out since the 1970s, including a larger share of women employed outside the home, more two-earner households, higher incomes, more affordable and convenient fast-food outlets, increased advertising by foodservice chains, and the smaller size of U.S. households (ERS 2014). The National Restaurant Association reported that in 1981 the average American ate 3.7 commercially prepared meals per week. By 2000, that number had increased to 4.2 per week. All those meals have contributed to the increase in overweight and obesity, as the frequency of eating in restaurants has been positively associated with body fatness. Ample evidence exists to show that, ounce for ounce, foods eaten away from home are more calorie-dense than foods prepared at home (McCrory et al. 1999). As the food service industry offers more choices, from fast food to a wide array of ethnic restaurants, the popularity of dining out implies that desire for convenience and variety overrides concern about obesity.

Physical Inactivity

Along with a growing tendency to consume more calories, Americans have become less active overall than they were 20 years ago. Given labor-saving devices, from personal automobiles to e-mail, and a technology-driven workforce that is shifting from physically demanding manual labor to sedentary work, we cannot expect daily caloric expenditure to increase. For most people, daily work no longer provides the opportunity for physical activity that it once did. As jobs have become more sedentary, the workweek has been expanding, so even less time is available for leisure-time physical activity.

The CDC and the Office of the Surgeon General recommend that all adults should do at least 30 minutes of moderate-intensity physical activity most days of the week. Activity does not need to be high intensity or done all at one time to be beneficial. An example of a moderate-intensity activity is brisk walking (a pace of 15–20 minutes per mile) for 30 minutes. The 30 minutes can be divided into three walks of 10 minutes each and still meet the recommendation (CDC 2008). National statistics from 2000 indicated that only about 20 percent of Americans reached the minimum activity goal. This percentage of inactive people had not changed since the 1970s, but during that period the population increased by about 60 million people, meaning that the number of sedentary Americans actually increased by 48 million. A 2014 CDC report indicated that less than half (48%) of all adults meet the U.S. Physical Activity Guidelines. Less than 3 in 10 high school students exercised enough to meet their recommendation of least 60 minutes of physical activity every day. Some groups are more physically active than others. Men (52.1%) are more likely than women (42.6%), and younger adults are more likely than older adults to meet the Guidelines for aerobic activity. Adults whose family income is above the poverty level are more likely to get enough physical activity than adults whose family income is at or near the poverty level (CDC 2014).

Due to the reduction of physical education in schools, the lack of access to playgrounds, and concerns for physical safety, many children do not get the recommended amount of daily activity. Researchers at Johns Hopkins University reported that watching television is the number one leisure-time activity among school-age children. A study from 1998 indicated that more than a quarter of U.S. children watch four or more hours of television a day (Andersen et al. 1998). A 2006 study reported that youth 6–13 years old spend approximately three hours per day watching television; however, when time spent on computers and video games is added, screen media exposure exceeds five hours per day (Jordan 2006). Television viewing affects childhood obesity in two ways: watching TV is sedentary, and food consumption is increased when children eat while viewing programs or as they respond to the frequent advertisements of high-calorie fun and exciting foods by reaching for more snacks (Powell et al. 2007).

Physical Activity and Short-Term Weight Loss

Physical activity has favorable effects on the body's metabolic systems, so numerous health benefits are gained from exercise even without weight loss. This point is important to keep in mind because, contrary to the belief that exercise causes weight loss, data from randomized controlled studies suggest that adding exercise to dietary therapy does not significantly increase short-term weight loss when compared with dieting without exercise (Wing 1999). Resistance exercise can build strength and muscle tissue, which may allow an obese or overweight person to become more physically active; however, neither resistance nor strength training increases weight loss (Jakicic et al. 2001,

2008). The ineffectiveness of moderate exercise alone to reduce body fat is not surprising when we consider that 1 pound of body fat contains the equivalent of about 3,500 Kcal, and to reduce body fat one must expend more energy than is taken in.

But moderate exercise is not useless. Depending on a person's body weight, 15 minutes of brisk walking uses about 100 Kcal. As shown in the list below, walking for 15 minutes seven days a week will theoretically result in only a 0.2-pound weight loss per week, but a 10-pound loss per year will be achieved if the walking is done every day and if food energy intake remains constant.

- A 15-minute brisk walk uses 100 Kcal of energy.
- 100 Kcal × 7 days = 700 Kcal deficit; 3,500 Kcal per pound of fat; 700/3,500 = 0.2 pound loss per week.
- Walking for 15 minutes seven days a week results in a 0.2-pound loss per week.
- Walking for 15 minutes 365 days a year results in a 10.4-pound loss per year.

Even though physical exercise does not contribute greatly to weight loss, it is absolutely necessary for weight maintenance and good health, and moderate exercise is an important factor in preventing regain after weight is lost.

The opportunity costs of being physically active during leisure time include time, effort, and sometimes money. The value of an alternate activity given up to spend time walking in the park has to be balanced with the health benefits. Costs to join a gym or health club or to purchase fitness equipment may be incurred. Health economists Darius Lakdawalla and Tomas Philipson noted that, in earlier agricultural and industrial times, energy expenditure was part of one's work and people were rewarded for their exercise. Today, physical labor is not always built into daily life, and people must spend time and money for exercise (Variyam 2005).

Metabolic and Genetic Contributions

Complex biological mechanisms involving fat cells, hormones, and neurochemical pathways in the brain regulate the balance between energy input and energy expenditure. Fat cells in the body serve two major functions: they store and release fatty acids ingested from food, and they secrete an array of biologically active molecules including the hormone leptin (Bray and Champagne 2005). Leptin, from the Greek word *leptos*, meaning thin, is a hormone produced by fat cells that are also called adipocytes. The hormone was discovered in the 1990s in genetically obese mice that carried the *ob* (obese) gene, which rendered them unable to make any leptin. Leptin thus regulates energy expenditure and food intake in rodents. As the amount of fat stored in adipocytes increases, leptin is released into the bloodstream and signals to the brain that the body has had enough to eat. Absolute leptin deficiency in humans, as in mice, causes severe obesity. These genetic defects are extremely rare in humans. Only about 10 children have been identified worldwide who have the disorder.

The discovery of the fat-regulating hormone was met with great hope that injecting patients with leptin could produce weight loss. However, clinical trials conducted in 1999 showed that, even with high doses of leptin, only a small amount of weight was lost. The results also demonstrated that most people with obesity already have high levels of leptin in their bloodstream. It was suggested that people with obesity are leptin resistant, and injecting more of the hormone simply has no effect (Heymsfield et al. 1999).

Information about hunger and satiety also comes from the gastrointestinal tract, where several peptides signal people and animals to stop or start eating. Ghrelin is one peptide that has received recent attention because, in contrast to other gastrointestinal hormones, it stimulates food intake (Cummings and Shannon 2003).

The brain is a major director in regulation of food intake. It receives and transmits information about hunger and satiety. An interesting discovery made in 2004 was that sleep deprivation enhances the release of peptides that produce hunger (Spiegel et al. 2004). In men, allowed to sleep only 4 hours per night for two days, leptin decreased and ghrelin increased when compared with the pattern seen in men who slept for 10 hours on each of the two nights. Is it possible that the epidemic of obesity may be a response to lack of sleep?

Can We Blame Obesity on Our Genes?

The role of genetic determinants of obesity, such as the *ob* gene and the hormone leptin as a modulator of food intake and energy expenditure, are intriguing, but they cannot explain the recent epidemic of obesity. Our human genome has not significantly changed in just a few decades. Genes themselves do not make a person obese or thin. They merely determine which individuals are susceptible to weight gain in response to environmental factors. Genetics loads the gun and the environment pulls the trigger.

Ways Genes Contribute to Obesity

Not all people exposed to an abundant food supply are obese. Furthermore, not all obese people exhibit adverse health consequences. This diversity occurs even among groups of the same racial or ethnic background and within families living in the same environment. The variation in how people respond to the same environmental conditions suggests that genes play a role. A common genetic explanation for the rapid rise in obesity is the "thrifty gene" hypothesis—the same genes that made it easier for our ancestors to survive occasional lack of food are now being challenged by environments in which food is always plentiful.

Ways that genes may influence individual propensity for obesity include poor regulation of appetite or the tendency to overeat, inclination to be sedentary or physically inactive, diminished metabolic ability to use dietary fats as fuel, and capacity to preferentially store body fat. The exact pathway by which these genes exert their effects and interact with environmental factors is unknown. Exploration of candidate genes through genomics (the study of genes, their molecular mechanisms, and their associations with health and disease) is an important area for future research regarding overweight and obesity. Use of family history is a straightforward way for clinicians and public health experts to reduce the impact of obesity now. Family history reflects the genetic background and environmental exposures shared by close relatives. Health care practitioners collect family health histories to identify people at high risk of obesity-related disorders such as diabetes, cardiovascular diseases, and some forms of cancer. Weight loss or prevention of excessive weight gain is especially important in this high-risk group. Although all people should follow a healthful diet and incorporate regular physical activity into their daily routine, health promotion programs to reduce disease associated with obesity are more effective if they are directed to the high-risk groups.

Clearly, some genetic factors influence excess weight gain. If weight control were simply a matter of willpower, obesity would not be a problem because few people would choose to be fat.

However, genes are not destiny. Obesity can be prevented or managed in most cases with a combination of diet, physical activity, behavior change, medication, or surgery. Finding the most effective combination of treatments for each individual is the challenge we now face.

Consequences of Overweight and Obesity

Although many Americans view overweight as a body image issue, the real concern is the extent to which overweight and obesity contribute directly to morbidity (disease or illness) and mortality (death) (Patel et al. 2006). A declaration from the Office of the Surgeon General of the United States says, "The primary concern of overweight and obesity is one of health and not appearance" (USDHHS 2007). As Hippocrates noted centuries ago, scientists today find that life expectancy is reduced by obesity. In 2003, before the U.S. House of Representatives,

Surgeon General Richard Carmona said, "I welcome this chance to talk with you about a health crisis affecting every State, every city, every community, and every school across our great Nation. The crisis is obesity. It's the fastest growing cause of death in America" (Carmona 2003).

Individuals who are obese (BMI ≥ 30) have a 10–50 percent increased risk of death from all causes compared with healthy-weight individuals (BMI 18.5–24.9), and the risk of death rises with increasing weight. Most of the increased deaths are due to cardiovascular causes (NHLBI 1998). Overweight and obesity increase risk for developing more than 35 major diseases, including heart disease; hypertension; type 2 diabetes; respiratory problems; osteoarthritis; gallbladder disease; and cancers of the endometrium, breast, prostate, and colon (NHLBI 1998). Obesity also has serious psychological consequences, such as low self-esteem and clinical depression (Kopelman 2000).

According to NHLBI (1998) report:

- The incidence of heart disease (heart attack, congestive heart failure, sudden cardiac death, and angina or chest pain) is increased in persons who have a BMI of 25 or greater.
- High blood pressure is twice as common in adults who are obese than in those who are at a healthy weight, and obesity is associated with elevated triglycerides (blood fat) and decreased HDL cholesterol ("good cholesterol").
- With a weight gain of 11–18 pounds, a person's risk of developing type 2 diabetes increases to twice that of individuals who have not gained weight. More than 80 percent of people with diabetes are overweight or obese.
- Sleep apnea (interrupted breathing while sleeping) is more common in obese persons. Obesity is associated with a higher prevalence of asthma.
- For every 2-pound increase in weight, the risk of developing arthritis is increased by 9–13 percent. Symptoms of arthritis often improve with weight loss.

Overweight and obesity are associated with an increased risk for some types of cancer, including endometrial (cancer of the lining of the uterus), colon, gallbladder, prostate, kidney, and breast cancer. Women who gain more than 20 pounds after age 18 double their risk of postmenopausal breast cancer, compared with women whose weight remains stable (NHLBI 1998).

Reproductive complications are increased with excess weight. Obesity during pregnancy is linked to increased risk of death in both the baby and the mother. The risk of maternal high blood pressure increases 10 times for overweight women. Women who are obese during pregnancy are more likely to have gestational diabetes (a form of type 2 diabetes that ceases when the baby is born). Women who are obese during pregnancy are more likely to have high–birth weight infants and may face a higher rate of cesarean section delivery. Obesity during pregnancy is associated with an increased risk of birth defects, including neural tube defects such as spina bifida.

A wide range of other physical and mental health consequences are related to excess weight. Overweight and obesity are associated with increased risks of gallbladder disease, incontinence, and complications during surgery. Obesity can affect quality of life by limiting mobility and decreasing physical endurance.

As little as 5–15 percent of total body weight loss in a person who is overweight or obese reduces the risk factors for some diseases, particularly heart disease and diabetes. Weight reduction is especially beneficial if a person has other risk factors, such as smoking, lack of physical activity, or a family history of heart disease (NHLBI 1998).

Discrimination

Obese individuals endure widespread stigma and discrimination in social, academic, and job situations. Negative perceptions of obese persons exist in the workplace. Research surveys indicated that co-workers and employers viewed obese employees as less competent and lacking in self-discipline. These attitudes can have a negative impact on wages, promotions, and hiring for obese employees. Other studies show that obese applicants are less likely to be hired than thinner applicants, despite having identical job qualifications (Brownell 2005).

Multiple forms of weight stigmatization occur in educational settings. Students with obesity face numerous obstacles, ranging from harassment to rejection by peers at school. Research shows that stigma toward overweight students begins early. Negative attitudes have been reported among preschool children (ages three to five), who said overweight peers were mean, stupid, ugly, unhappy, and lazy and had few friends (Puhl and Brownell 2001).

Weight stigma also exists in health care settings. Obese patients may be reluctant to seek medical care and are more likely to delay important preventive health care services and cancel medical appointments to avoid experiencing weight bias from health care providers. Negative attitudes about overweight patients have been reported by physicians, nurses, dietitians, psychologists, and medical students. Evidence exists that even health care professionals who specialize in the treatment of obesity hold negative attitudes (Schwartz et al. 2003).

Taken together, the consequences of being denied jobs, rejected by peers, or treated inappropriately by health care professionals because of one's weight can have a serious and negative impact on quality of life. This effect can lead to a number of psychological problems that add to physical difficulties. Obesity-related mental health disorders include depression, anxiety, and despair. Given the pervasive nature of weight stigma in U.S. society, transforming attitudes and enforcing laws that prohibit discrimination based on weight are necessary to decrease the problem of bias against obese individuals. To further this aim, Dr. Rebecca Puhl, Deputy Director at the Rudd Center for Food Policy & Obesity, is responsible for research and policy efforts aimed at reducing weight bias. She states that "Stigmatization of obese individuals threatens health, generates health disparities, and interferes with effective obesity intervention efforts" (Puhl 2010).

Economic Consequences

Obesity has a clearly measurable impact on physical and mental health, health-related quality of life, and generates considerable direct and indirect costs (Dixon 2010). Both direct and indirect health care costs are increased. Direct health care costs refer to preventive, diagnostic, and treatment services, such as physician visits, medications, and hospital and nursing home care. Indirect costs occur when people are unable to work because of illness or disability, and thus do not receive wages (Colditz 1999).

Studies to determine costs of obesity have shown that health care expenditure among both underweight and overweight individuals increase as BMI varies from the healthy weight range. An analysis of more than 16,000 individuals using data from the 1987 National Medical Expenditure Survey confirmed that BMI, either higher or lower than the healthy weight range of normal, was related to increased medical expenditures (Heithoff et al. 1997; Finkelstein et al. 2005).

In 1998, the medical costs of obesity were estimated to be as high as $78.5 billion, with roughly half financed by Medicare and Medicaid. A study of medical spending through 2006 indicated that obesity costs were responsible for almost $40 billion (Finkelstein 2009). Other studies indicated that increased health care expenditures were largely related to such costly chronic medical conditions as diabetes and hypertension. Studies from Kaiser Permanente, a large national health maintenance organization, support the BMI and health cost relationship (Thompson et al. 2001). According to one Kaiser analysis of more than 17,000 patients, total excess costs to the health plan from obese participants amounted to $220 million, or about 6 percent of total expenses for all plan members (Quesenberry, Caan, and Jacobson 1998). Costs were increased among obese members for pharmacy services, outpatient services, and inpatient care.

The significant increase in numbers of extremely obese patients (BMI $\geq$ 40) puts additional strains on the health care system. Lifting injuries among physical therapists, nurses, and other health care workers are common. New hospital expenditures are required for special beds, scales, operating tables, and wheelchairs that will accommodate the weight of very heavy patients.

The costs of obesity treatment must be balanced with predicted outcomes. A weight loss of as little as 5 percent produces health benefits such as lowering blood pressure, blood sugar, and triglycerides (the form in which fat is carried in the blood). Such health improvements could offset the costs of obesity therapy over the long term (NHLBI 1998). However, even after weight loss, formerly obese people need routine follow-up, as with control of other chronic conditions such as diabetes. Another factor to be weighed is cost reimbursement. Without adequate reimbursement, physicians are hesitant to take on long-term patient obesity management. Some health insurers cover obesity treatment, but the coverage is not widespread. A key question is: will a large investment in developing and implementing effective obesity treatment and prevention produce a sufficient increase in good health, happiness, and longevity and a decrease in health care costs?

We Live in an Obesogenic Environment

Although one individual might be born with a stronger tendency to gain weight than another, certain circumstances also must be in place to facilitate weight gain. An environment conducive to weight gain has been termed "obesogenic" (Swinburn, Egger, and Raza 1999). Three primary environmental factors of the obesogenic environment contribute to overweight and obesity:

- Eating more food than the body can use
- Too little exercise or activity
- Lifestyles that interfere with healthy eating and activity (Galvez, Frieden, and Landrigan 2003)

The current situation in the United States encourages energy consumption and discourages energy expenditure to the point that people, who could have maintained a healthy weight in the past decades, find it too difficult to do so today. Americans have easy access to a wide variety of good-tasting, inexpensive, calorie-rich foods that are served and marketed in increasingly large portions. Food is everywhere. It can be found in convenience stores, vending machines, gas stations, museums, and even libraries. The fast-food industry provides a combination of convenience, large portions, and low cost. These factors are attractive to many Americans (Variyam 2005).

On the energy output side, increasing numbers of Americans lead essentially sedentary lives. Many people sit all day at computers and use cars to get to and from work. Even leisure time is spent in sedentary activities such as watching television and shopping, communicating, or playing games on a computer.

The obesity epidemic is a result of these interacting issues. The solution lies in changing them at individual, community, governmental, and cultural levels. Interventions that have been suggested to help prevent obesity include mass media campaigns, increased availability of exercise opportunities, taxes on high-fat and high-sugar foods, control of food advertising during children's television programming, and restoration of daily physical activity in schools.

Each intervention has positive and negative aspects that may create conflict and controversy. The following chapters will present issues that frame debates about the causes, assessment, treatment, and prevention of obesity. These explanations and findings are based on scientific research that uncovers answers to current concerns about obesity, including the true impact of an obesogenic environment, the merit of various diets, medications or surgeries, and even the stance that obesity may not actually be a public crisis that requires intervention.

References

American College of Sports Medicine (ACSM). *ACSM's Resource Manual for Guidelines for Exercise Testing and Prescription*. 4th ed. Baltimore: Lippincott Williams & Wilkins, 2001.

American Heart Association (AHA). *A Nation at Risk: Obesity in the United States, a Statistical Sourcebook.* Dallas: American Heart Association and the Robert Wood Johnson Foundation, 2005.

Andersen, R. E., C. J. Crespo, S. J. Bartlett, L. J. Cheskin, and M. Pratt. "Relationship of Physical Activity and Television Watching with Body Weight and Level of Fatness among Children: Results from the Third National Health and Nutrition Examination Survey." *Journal of the American Medical Association* 279, no. 12 (1998): 938–942.

Banting, W. *Letter on Corpulence, Addressed to the Public.* London: Harrison, 1864.

Bolanowski, M., and B. E. Nilsson. "Assessment of Human Body Composition Using Dual-Energy X-Ray Absorptiometry and Bioelectrical Impedance Analysis." *Medical Science Monitor* 7, no. 5 (2001): 1029–1033.

Bray, G. A., and C. M. Champagne. "Beyond Energy Balance: There Is More to Obesity Than Kilocalories." *Journal of the American Dietetic Association* 105, no. 5, Suppl. 1 (2005): S17–S23.

Breslow, L. "Public Health Aspects of Weight Control." *American Journal of Public Health and the Nation's Health* 42, no. 9 (1952): 1116–1120.

Brownell, K. D. "The Chronicling of Obesity: Growing Awareness of Its Social, Economic, and Political Contexts." *Journal of Health Politics, Policy and Law* 30, no. 5 (2005): 955–964.

Carmona, R. "The Obesity Crisis in America." In Testimony before the Subcommittee on Education Reform Committee on Education and the Workforce United States House of Representatives, edited by Surgeon General, U.S. Public Health Service. Washington, DC: U.S. Department of Health and Human Services, 2003.

Centers for Disease Control and Prevention (CDC). "About BMI for Children and Teens." Page last updated:

September 3, 2014. Accessed January 15, 2015. http://www.cdc.gov/obesity/data/childhood.html.

Centers for Disease Control and Prevention (CDC). "Adult Obesity Facts." Page last updated: September 9, 2014. Accessed January 15, 2015. http://www.cdc.gov/obesity/data/adult.html.

Centers for Disease Control and Prevention (CDC). "Anthropometric Reference Data, United States, 1988–1994." 1999. Accessed February 5, 2008. http://www.cdc.gov/nchs/about/major/nhanes/anthropometric_measures.htm.

Centers for Disease Control and Prevention (CDC). "Facts about Physical Activity." Page last updated: May 23, 2014. Accessed December 10, 2014. http://www.cdc.gov/physicalactivity/data/facts.html.

Centers for Disease Control and Prevention (CDC). "Final Review, Healthy People 2010: Nutrition and Overweight." January 2013. Accessed January 15, 2015. http://www.cdc.gov/nchs/data/hpdata2010/hp2010_final_review_focus_area_19.pdf.

Centers for Disease Control and Prevention (CDC). "Obesity Prevalence Maps." Page last updated: September 9, 2014. Accessed January 15, 2015. http://www.cdc.gov/obesity/data/prevalence-maps.html.

Centers for Disease Control and Prevention (CDC). "Portion Size: Then and Now." 2006. Accessed January 5, 2009. http://www.cdc.gov/nccdphp/dnpa/nutrition/pdf/portion_size_research.pdf.

Colditz, G. A. "Economic Costs of Obesity and Inactivity." *Medicine & Science in Sports & Exercise* 31, no. 11, Suppl. (1999): S663–S667.

Cummings, D. E., and M. H. Shannon. "Roles for Ghrelin in the Regulation of Appetite and Body Weight." *Archives of Surgery* 138, no. 4 (2003): 389–396.

DiMeglio, D. P., and R. D. Mattes. "Liquid versus Solid Carbohydrate: Effects on Food Intake and Body Weight." *International Journal of Obesity and Related Metabolic Disorders* 24, no. 6 (2000): 794–800.

Dixon, J. B. "The Effect of Obesity on Health Outcomes." *Molecular and Cellular Endocrinology* 316, no. 2 (2010): 104–108.

ERS. USDA Economic Research Service. "Food-Away-from-Home." Last updated: Wednesday, October 29, 2014. Accessed December 15, 2015. http://www.ers.usda.gov/topics/food-choices-health/food-consumption-demand/food-away-from-home.aspx.

Erselcan, T., F. Candan, S. Saruhan, and T. Ayca. "Comparison of Body Composition Analysis Methods in Clinical Routine." *Annals of Nutrition and Metabolism* 44, no. 5–6 (2000): 243–248.

Finkelstein, E. A., C. J. Ruhm, and K. M. Kosa. "Economic Causes and Consequences of Obesity." *Annual Review of Public Health*, 26 (2005): 239–257.

Finkelstein, E. A., J. G. Trogdon, J. W. Cohen, and W. Dietz. "Annual Medical Spending Attributable to Obesity: Payer-and Service-Specific Estimates." *Health Affairs (Millwood)* 28, no. 5 (2009): w822–w831.

Fisher, J. O., Y. Liu, L. L. Birch, and B. J. Rolls. "Effects of Portion Size and Energy Density on Young Children's Intake at a Meal." *American Journal of Clinical Nutrition* 86, no. 1 (2007): 174–179.

Flegal, K. M., B. I. Graubard, D. F. Williamson, and M. H. Gail. "Excess Deaths Associated with Underweight, Overweight, and Obesity." *Journal of the American Medical Association* 293, no. 15 (2005): 1861–1867.

Flegal, K. M., M. D. Carroll, C. L. Ogden, and L. R. Curtin. "Prevalence and Trends in Obesity among U.S. Adults,

1999–2008." *Journal of the American Medical Association* 303, no. 3 (2010): 235–241.

Ford, E. S., A. H. Mokdad, and W. H. Giles. "Trends in Waist Circumference among U.S. Adults." *Obesity Research* 11, no. 10 (2003): 1223–1231.

Franklin, B. "Poor Richard, an Almanack for 1737." Accessed January 5, 2009. http://www.vlib.us/amdocs/index.html.

Fryar, C. "Prevalence of Overweight, Obesity, and Extreme Obesity among Adults: United States, 1960–1962 through 2011–2012." Division of Health and Nutrition Examination Surveys. Page last updated: September 19, 2014. Accessed January 10, 2015. http://www.cdc. gov/nchs/data/hestat/obesity_adult_11_12/obesity_ adult_11_12.htm.

Gallagher, D. "Overweight and Obesity BMI Cut-offs and Their Relation to Metabolic Disorders in Koreans/Asians." *Obesity Research* 12, no. 3 (2004): 440–441.

Galvez, M. P., T. R. Frieden, and P. J. Landrigan. "Obesity in the 21st Century." *Environmental Health Perspectives* 111, no. 13 (2003): A684–A685.

Goran, M. I. "Energy Metabolism and Obesity." *Medical Clinics of North America* 84, no. 2 (2000): 347–362.

Guthrie, J. F., B. H. Lin, and E. Frazao. "Role of Food Prepared Away from Home in the American Diet, 1977–78 versus 1994–96: Changes and Consequences." *Journal of Nutrition Education and Behavior* 34, no. 3 (2002): 140–150.

Guthrie, J. F., and J. F. Morton. "Food Sources of Added Sweeteners in the Diets of Americans." *Journal of the American Dietetic Association* 100, no. 1 (2000): 43–51; quiz 49–50.

Hamwi, G. J. "Therapy: Changing Dietary Concepts." In *Diabetes Mellitus: Diagnosis and Treatment*, edited by T.S. Danowski, 73–78. New York: American Diabetes Association, 1964.

Heithoff, K. A., B. J. Cuffel, S. Kennedy, and J. Peters. "The Association between Body Mass and Health Care Expenditures." *Clinical Therapeutics* 19, no. 4 (1997): 811–820.

Heymsfield, S. B., A. S. Greenberg, K. Fujioka, R. M. Dixon, R. Kushner, T. Hunt, J. A. Lubina, J. Patane, B. Self, P. Hunt, and M. McCamish. "Recombinant Leptin for Weight Loss in Obese and Lean Adults: A Randomized, Controlled, Dose-Escalation Trial." *Journal of the American Medical Association* 282, no. 16 (1999): 1568–1575.

Heymsfield, S. B., Z. Wang, M. Visser, D. Gallagher, and R. N. Pierson, Jr. "Techniques Used in the Measurement of Body Composition: An Overview with Emphasis on Bioelectrical Impedance Analysis." *American Journal of Clinical Nutrition* 64, no. 3, Suppl. (1996): 478S–484S.

Jakicic, J. M., K. Clark, E. Coleman, J. E. Donnelly, J. Foreyt, E. Melanson, J. Volek, and S. L. Volpe. "American College of Sports Medicine Position Stand. Appropriate Intervention Strategies for Weight Loss and Prevention of Weight Regain for Adults." *Medicine & Science in Sports & Exercise* 33, no. 12 (2001): 2145–2156.

Jakicic, J. M., B. H. Marcus, W. Lang, and C. Janney. "Effect of Exercise on 24-Month Weight Loss Maintenance in Overweight Women." *Archives of Internal Medicine* 168, no. 14 (2008): 1550–1559; discussion 1559–1560.

Johnson, L., A. P. Mander, L. R. Jones, P. M. Emmett, and S. A. Jebb. "Is Sugar-Sweetened Beverage Consumption Associated with Increased Fatness in Children?" *Nutrition* 23, no. 7–8 (2007): 557–563.

Jordan, A. B., J. C. Hersey, J. A. McDivitt, C. D. Heitzler. "Reducing Children's Television-Viewing Time: a Qualitative Study of Parents and Their Children." *Pediatrics* 118, no. 5 (2006): e1303–e1310.

Kopelman, P. G. "Obesity as a Medical Problem." *Nature* 404, no. 6778 (2000): 635–643.

Kuczmarski, R. J., and K. M. Flegal. "Criteria for Definition of Overweight in Transition: Background and Recommendations for the United States." *American Journal of Clinical Nutrition* 72, no. 5 (2000): 1074–1081.

Luciano, Lynne. *Looking Good: Male Body Image in Modern America.* New York: Hill and Wang, 2001.

McCrory, M. A., P. J. Fuss, N. P. Hays, A. G. Vinken, A. S. Greenberg, and S. B. Roberts. "Overeating in America: Association between Restaurant Food Consumption and Body Fatness in Healthy Adult Men and Women Ages 19 to 80." *Obesity Research* 7, no. 6 (1999): 564–751.

Metropolitan Life Insurance Company (MLIC). "Metropolitan Life Insurance Company. Ideal Weights for Men 1942." *Statistical Bulletin–Metropolitan Life Insurance Company* 23 (1942): 6–8.

Metropolitan Life Insurance Company (MLIC). "Metropolitan Life Insurance Company. Ideal Weights for Women." *Statistical Bulletin–Metropolitan Life Insurance Company* 24 (1943): 6–8.

Metropolitan Life Insurance Company (MLIC). "New Weight Standards for Men and Women." *Statistical Bulletin–Metropolitan Life Insurance Company* 40 (1959): 1–10.

Metropolitan Life Insurance Company (MLIC). "1983 Metropolitan Height and Weight Tables: New York." *Statistical Bulletin–Metropolitan Life Insurance Company* 64 (1983): 6–8.

Miller, P. E., J. Reedy, S. I. Kirkpatrick, and S. M. Krebs-Smith. "The United States Food Supply Is Not Consistent with Dietary Guidance: Evidence from an Evaluation Using the Healthy Eating Index-2010." *Journal of the Academy of Nutrition and Dietetics* 115, no. 1 (2015): 95–100.

MMWR. Morbidity and Mortality Weekly Report. "Sugar-Sweetened Beverage Consumption Among Adults—18 States, 2012." August 15, 2014, 63(32); 686–690. Accessed December 15, 2014. http://www.cdc .gov/mmwr/preview/mmwrhtml/mm6332a2.htm.

National Center for Health Statistics (NCHS). "Chartbook on Trends in the Health of Americans. Health, United States, 2006." Washington, DC: U.S. Public Health Service, 2006.

National Heart, Lung and Blood Institute (NHLBI). Clinical Guidelines on the Identification, Evaluation, and Treatment of Overweight and Obesity in Adults: The Evidence Report. Bethesda, MD: National Heart, Lung and Blood Institute, 1998.

National Institutes of Health (NIH). "Clinical Guidelines on the Identification, Evaluation, and Treatment of Overweight and Obesity in Adults—the Evidence Report. National Institutes of Health." *Obesity Research* 6, Suppl. 2 (1998): 51S–209S.

Nestle, M., and M. F. Jacobson. "Halting the Obesity Epidemic: A Public Health Policy Approach." *Public Health Reports* 115, no. 1 (2000): 12–24.

Nielsen, S. J., and B. M. Popkin. "Patterns and Trends in Food Portion Sizes, 1977–1998." *Journal of the American Medical Association* 289, no. 4 (2003): 450–453.

The Obesity Society. "Obesity Statistics." Accessed January 15, 2015. http://www.obesity.org/resources-for/ obesity-statistics.htm.

Ogden, C. L., M. D. Carroll, B. K. Kit, and K. M. Flegal. "Prevalence of Childhood and Adult Obesity in the United States, 2011–2012." *Journal of the American Medical Association* 311, no. 8 (2014): 806–814.

Olshansky, S. J., D. J. Passaro, R. C. Hershow, J. Layden, B. A. Carnes, J. Brody, L. Hayflick, R. N. Butler, D. B. Allison, and D. S. Ludwig. "A Potential Decline in Life

Expectancy in the United States in the 21st Century." *New England Journal of Medicine* 352, no. 11 (2005): 1138–1145.

Patel, M. R., M. Donahue, P. W. Wilson, and R. M. Califf. "Clinical Trial Issues in Weight-Loss Therapy." *American Heart Journal* 151, no. 3 (2006): 633–642.

Powell, L. M., G. Szczypka, F. J. Chaloupka, and C. L. Braunschweig. "Nutritional Content of Television Food Advertisements Seen by Children and Adolescents in the United States." *Pediatrics* 120, no. 3 (2007): 576–583.

Puhl, R., and K. D. Brownell. "Bias, Discrimination, and Obesity." *Obesity Research* 9, no. 12 (2001): 788–805.

Puhl, R. M., and C. A. Heuer. "Obesity Stigma: Important Considerations for Public Health." *American Journal of Public Health* 100, no. 6 (2010): 1019–1028.

Putnam, J., L. S. Kantor, and J. Allshouse. "Per Capita Food Supply Trends: Progress toward Dietary Guidelines." *Food Review* 23 (2000): 2–14.

Quesenberry, C. P., Jr., B. Caan, and A. Jacobson. "Obesity, Health Services Use, and Health Care Costs among Members of a Health Maintenance Organization." *Archives of Internal Medicine* 158, no. 5 (1998): 466–472.

Razak, F., S. S. Anand, H. Shannon, V. Vuksan, B. Davis, R. Jacobs, K. K. Teo, M. McQueen, and S. Yusuf. "Defining Obesity Cut Points in a Multiethnic Population." *Circulation* 115, no. 16 (2007): 2111–2118.

Rolls, B. J., E. L. Morris, and L. S. Roe. "Portion Size of Food Affects Energy Intake in Normal-Weight and Overweight Men and Women." *American Journal of Clinical Nutrition* 76, no. 6 (2002): 1207–1213.

Schwartz, M. B., H. O. Chambliss, K. D. Brownell, S. N. Blair, and C. Billington. "Weight Bias among Health Professionals Specializing in Obesity." *Obesity Research* 11, no. 9 (2003): 1033–1039.

Spiegel, K., E. Tasali, P. Penev, and E. Van Cauter. "Brief Communication: Sleep Curtailment in Healthy Young Men Is Associated with Decreased Leptin Levels, Elevated Ghrelin Levels, and Increased Hunger and Appetite." *Annals of Internal Medicine* 141, no. 11 (2004): 846–850.

Swinburn, B., G. Egger, and F. Raza. "Dissecting Obesogenic Environments: The Development and Application of a Framework for Identifying and Prioritizing Environmental Interventions for Obesity." *Preventive Medicine* 29, no. 6, Pt. 1 (1999): 563–570.

Symonds, Brandreth. "The Influence of Overweight and Underweight on Vitality." *A Weekly Journal of Medicine and Surgery* 74 (1908): 389–393.

Thompson, D., J. B. Brown, G. A. Nichols, P. J. Elmer, and G. Oster. "Body Mass Index and Future Healthcare Costs: A Retrospective Cohort Study." *Obesity Research* 9, no. 3 (2001): 210–218.

U.S. Department of Health and Human Services (USDHHS). "Overweight and Obesity: Health Consequences." Washington, DC: USHHS, 2007.

U.S. Department of Health and Human Services (USDHHS). "The Surgeon General's Call to Action to Prevent and Decrease Overweight and Obesity." Washington, DC: USHHS, 2001.

U.S. Department of Health and Human Services (USDHHS). "Healthy People 2020." Washington, DC. Site last updated November 30, 2014. Accessed December 15, 2014. http://www.healthypeople.gov/.

Variyam, Jayachandran N. "The Price Is Right: Economics and the Rise in Obesity." *Amber Waves* February (2005): 21–27.

Wang, J., J. C. Thornton, S. Kolesnik, and R. N. Pierson, Jr. "Anthropometry in Body Composition. An Overview."

Annals of the New York Academy of Sciences 904 (2000): 317–326.

Wansink, B., and J. Kim. "Bad Popcorn in Big Buckets: Portion Size Can Influence Intake as Much as Taste." *Journal of Nutrition Education and Behavior* 37, no. 5 (2005): 242–245.

Weight-control Information Network (WIN). "Understanding Adult Obesity." 2006. Accessed January 5, 2009. http://win.niddk.nih.gov/publications/understanding.htm.

Wing, R. R. "Physical Activity in the Treatment of the Adulthood Overweight and Obesity: Current Evidence and Research Issues." *Medicine & Science in Sports & Exercise* 31, no. 11, Suppl. (1999): S547–S552.

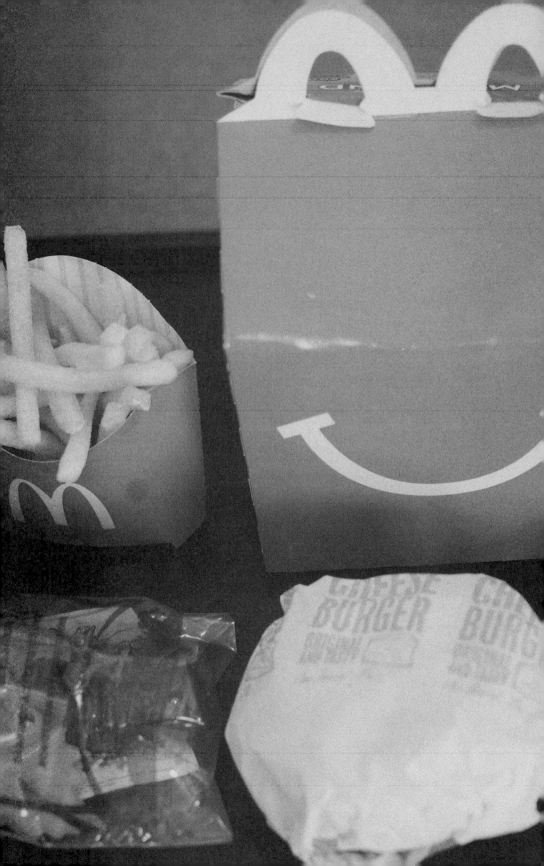

2 Problems, Controversies, and Solutions

Introduction

The problems, controversies, and solutions discussed in this chapter have been debated by researchers, health care professionals, and policy makers for decades. Is obesity a disease or is it a moral failing? Can obesity be called an epidemic? How should obesity be treated? What are the public health aspects and responsibilities? The answers to these questions are not simple and have major implications for U.S. society and its health care system.

Is Obesity a Disease?

Advocates of defining obesity as a disease contend that this label will allow the condition to be taken more seriously. Those opposed to calling obesity a disease say it will override personal and societal responsibility. Although not without controversy, increasing scientific evidence and medical consensus support the disease designation. It is generally accepted that a disease must have at least two of the following three features: (1) recognized etiologic agents, (2) identifiable signs and symptoms,

McDonald's Happy Meals are marketed as explicitly for children and the meals often also include popular small toys. Because prevention of child obesity is an important public health issue, food offerings geared to children should encourage healthier dietary choices. As a response to health-minded parents, in 2015, McDonald's offered a Chicken McNugget Happy Meal that included kids' size portions of McNuggets made with white meat, french fries, and a choice of apple slices or low-fat strawberry yogurt. (AP Photo/Eric Risberg)

and (3) consistent anatomical alterations. Obesity meets all three criteria.

First, the recognized etiologic (causative) agents are a combination of metabolic, physiologic, genetic, social, behavioral, and cultural factors. Second, some identifiable signs and symptoms include an excess accumulation of fat tissue as well as increased risk of breathing problems (sleep apnea), high blood glucose (type 2 diabetes), and high blood pressure (hypertension). Third, the consistent anatomic alteration is a body composition with a high percentage of body fat. Behaviors such as overeating or lack of exercise are not part of the definition of obesity. In 1985, the National Institutes of Health (NIH) declared that obesity met the definition of a disease based on studies showing that specific biochemical alterations occur in humans and experimental animals in response to environmental agents.

Doctors and scientists who say obesity should be labeled as a disease point to its link with increased morbidity and mortality. Physicians who specialize in endocrinology, family practice, and bariatrics (treatment of obesity) accept that obesity is a disease. When classified a disease, obesity research scientists may receive funding to develop effective interventions. Patients are able to get the treatment they need, and third-party payers pay for weight reduction services. Physicians have complained that obesity screening, weight management care, and counseling services are difficult to code for payment. Without proper coding, they cannot bill for obesity; rather, they have to bill for osteoarthritis, hypertension, diabetes, or other conditions that may exist as a side effect of obesity.

Reimbursement for obesity treatment got support in 2002 when the Internal Revenue Service (IRS) recognized obesity as a disease and allowed payments for medically valid obesity treatments to be claimed as a medical tax deduction (IRS 2002). This decision helped to legitimize the possibility of coverage from government and private insurers. In 2004, U.S. Department of Health and Human Services (HHS) Secretary Tommy Thompson and Medicare administrator Mark McClellan announced that the phrase "Obesity itself cannot be considered an illness" was removed from regulations that guide payment for medical treatment (HHS 2004). However, the wording change did not authorize any coverage for new treatments. For obesity to be recognized and covered, the provider was required to supply scientific evidence that a treatment works to improve Medicare beneficiaries' health outcomes. In other words, practitioners and government and industry partners who believe that obesity is an actual disease are responsible for collecting data from clinical trials on the effectiveness of proposed treatments. The federal government led the way again in 2014 when the Office of Personnel Management, which governs federal employee health benefits, announced that federal insurance plans may not deny coverage of Food and Drug Administration (FDA)-approved weight loss medications. The announcement noted that obesity could not be considered a "lifestyle" condition or that weight loss treatment was "cosmetic" (Dea 2014). This move by the U.S. government could encourage commercial insurance providers to also cover weight loss medications in their plans.

Current understanding is that the genetic tendency to obesity is both metabolic and behavioral. Obesity occurs as the result of disturbances in the way energy is stored or expended and of biologically driven abnormalities in appetite, satiation, and satiety. Independent of willpower, a person with one of these disturbances may never be satisfied after eating. Genes, and not personal control, may ultimately determine how much a person eats. Leanness or fatness may simply be a genetic trait.

Skeptical opponents of calling obesity a disease offer other explanations. They assert that obesity-associated disorders are not necessarily caused by increased body weight. Rather, they propose that a particular disease or treatment for disease may actually promote obesity. These skeptics point to the example of type 2 diabetes, a disorder that currently seems to pose the biggest threat to public health, in that some diabetes medications and strict blood sugar management cause weight gain. Compared with 35 percent prevalence of obesity in the general population, the Centers for Disease Control and Prevention (CDC) reports that 55 percent of adults with diabetes are obese. As obesity has become more prevalent, so has diabetes. What is the cause, and what is the effect? Does obesity cause diabetes, for example, or does diabetes lead to obesity? Poor health consequences may occur in obese people because they are more likely to belong to an unhealthy group—one that is older or has low socioeconomic status—or to an ethnic minority that has an increased risk for disease in individuals of all weights. Others suggest that it is hazardous weight loss practices and repeated loss and regain of weight that is the major contributor to obesity-related disease (Ernsberger 1989).

Opponents to the disease designation further contend that not all obese people are unhealthy and that calling obesity a medical problem reduces individual responsibility for taking ownership for lifestyle habits and maintaining a healthy weight. Even when people have a genetic tendency to gain weight, overeating and inactivity are the main causes of obesity. The gene pool has not changed, but eating habits have. Some physicians who work with obesity issues believe that, while obesity is a serious problem, it is not a disease in its own right. They say that when obesity is considered a disease it implies that individuals have no control over what is happening to their weight and health. Even though the debate continues, in 2013 the members of the American Medical Association (AMA) approved a policy that labeled obesity as a disease that requires a range of medical interventions (Breymaier 2013). Despite growing evidence for the benefit of providing lifestyle interventions, pharmacotherapy, and bariatric surgery for the treatment of obesity, survey data suggest that only a minority of clinicians actually provide such care (Kushner 2014).

Debate also surrounds how the disease label will affect individual patients with regard to stigma. Proponents maintain that diagnosing obesity as a serious disease removes the stigma associated with extra body fat. Those opposed argue that the disease designation actually further stigmatizes people who do not feel sick and do not notice any ill effects from extra weight. This line of thinking underscores one of the problems surrounding efforts to address obesity: An unhealthy diet and a sedentary lifestyle are health risks for anyone—fat or lean. Thus, those opposed to the disease label are concerned that reclassifying obesity as a disease places too much emphasis on the number on the scale and neglects the importance of a healthful lifestyle. As even the best weight loss interventions have limited efficacy, telling a patient to lose weight generally results in frustration and guilt. Many clinicians propose alternative strategies such as encouraging the individual to eat more fruits and vegetables, to get adequate sleep, and to enjoyable physical activity. These changes might actually prolong and improve life for all sizes.

Defining obesity as a disease may put too much emphasis on the medical aspect when every institution and individual involved should accept some responsibility. A number of businesses are taking on that responsibility. Food companies are pledging to make healthier snacks. Fast food chains promise new low-fat choices. Employers are integrating health management options such as gyms, diet groups, cafeterias with healthful foods, and health screening right at the work site. Health plans and doctors are initiating new prevention, treatment, and weight management programs. Local communities are constructing more walking and bike trails and after-school-activity programs for children.

In summing up the pros and cons of whether obesity is a disease, those who agree say:

- Obesity is linked to increased morbidity and mortality.
- Everyone would take the condition more seriously.
- There could be better reimbursement for medical treatment.
- Obese people would not be stigmatized as lacking willpower.

Those who disagree say:

- It would reduce the importance of individual responsibility.
- It would place too much emphasis on medical interventions.

- It would put undue social pressure and stigma on obese people who are healthy.
- The evidence is not sufficient to implicate obesity as a risk factor in its own right (Stagg-Elliott 2006).

Is Obesity an Epidemic?

A public opinion survey found that 85 percent of Americans believe that obesity is an epidemic and that the government should have a role in tackling the obesity crisis (Levi 2007). In 2001, U.S. Surgeon General David Satcher declared that obesity was reaching epidemic proportions and could soon be the cause of as much preventable disease and death as cigarette smoking. He released a call to action to promote the recognition of obesity as a health problem and to develop programs to treat obesity and encourage people to change their eating and exercise habits. But even with the urging of America's top physician, obesity statistics did not improve and the rate of overweight and obesity kept growing. In 2003, Surgeon General Richard H. Carmona spoke about the obesity crisis in the United States: "It is the fastest-growing cause of disease and death in America. And it is completely preventable. Nearly two out of every three Americans are overweight or obese. One out of every eight deaths in America is caused by an illness directly related to overweight and obesity" (Carmona 2003).

"Epidemic" is an emotionally charged term. It has different meanings for different people. For the general public, it is associated with a rapidly spreading and uncontrolled disease. Professional health researchers may use the term quite differently. Epidemiologists define an epidemic as the occurrence in a specified area of an illness or other health-related events in excess of what would normally be expected. Disease and epidemics occur as a result of the interaction of three factors: agent, host, and environment. Agents (too much food) cause the disease (extra body fat), hosts are genetically susceptible, and environmental conditions (easy access to high-calorie foods and reduced need to be active) permit host exposure to the agent. Understanding interactions between agent, host, and environment is crucial for discovering the best ways to prevent or control the spread of obesity.

The Center for Consumer Freedom (CFF) is a nonprofit organization of restaurants, food companies, and consumers. Its stated goal is to promote personal responsibility and protect consumer choice. The group has published a response to the description of obesity as an epidemic entitled "An Epidemic of Obesity Myths" (CFF 2004). It says the epidemic is a myth because, while more people are heavier than ever, the figures used to calculate the number of deaths attributed to obesity are flawed and the health risks of moderate obesity have been greatly overstated. The Center also contends that better diagnosis and treatment of high cholesterol and blood pressure have more than compensated for any increases in mortality from rising obesity. CCF may not have been too far off the mark when it pointed out problems with past statistical estimations of obesity increased risk of death. In 2005, Dr. Katherine Flegal, a researcher at the CDC, revised estimates of the deaths due to obesity after it became clear that previous measurement methods were out of date. An estimate, published in the *Journal of the American Medical Association*, showed that people in the overweight category, with a body mass index (BMI) of 25–29.9, typically live longer than normal-weight people, who have a BMI of 18–24.9 (Flegal 2005). Flegal and colleagues reported that the number of obesity-related deaths is significantly lower than previously believed. When National Health and Nutrition Examination Surveys (NHANES) data, which measured weights, heights, and death from 1988 to 2000, were analyzed, even severe obesity failed to appear as a statistically significant mortality risk.

More than a dozen other studies came to the same conclusion. Epidemiological analyses revealed that, aside from the extremes, BMI is not a strong predictor of death rates. The minimum risk for mortality seems to be associated with a BMI of approximately 25. The risk of death increases or decreases on upper or lower side of 25, respectively. In a study of nearly 10,000 older adults BMI trajectories, changes is weight over time were more predictive of mortality risk than initial BMI status. People in the overweight and stable trajectory had the highest survival rate (Zheng 2013).

Flegal's group speculates that, in recent decades, improvements in medical care have reduced the mortality level associated with obesity (Flegal 2005). This speculation is supported by research (also based on NHANES data) showing, in spite of increases in overweight and obesity, significant declines in high blood pressure, high cholesterol, and smoking. These are all risk factors for cardiovascular disease. Importantly, the greatest improvements occurred in the heaviest people (Gregg 2005). Although Americans are heavier than ever, they are also healthier than they were in the 1960s and 1970s. The average BMI was lower in those days, but the rate of deaths from cancer and heart disease was higher. In short, people live longer now (Kochanek 2014). Even though the CDC findings, reported widely in the media, caused confusion and questions about whether obesity really was a problem, some facts about obesity are not disputed. The proportion of the population that is overweight or obese continues to rise rapidly. Despite debates about obesity as a cause of death, there is little argument about the significant impact it has as a cause of disease. Excess weight is known to be a major contributor to diabetes, cardiovascular diseases, arthritis, and some forms of cancer. Even if obesity does cause fewer deaths than have previously been reported, it continues to be a serious public health problem.

An interesting addition to the discussion about whether obesity is an epidemic was published in the *New England Journal of Medicine*. The researchers suggested that obesity is influenced by one's social network and that it is "socially contagious." To see if obesity really did behave like an epidemic, they studied the effects of these groups on obesity. They examined data from the Framingham Heart Study—a very large social network that involves 12,000 people, including family, friends, and neighbors who have been studied and followed for more than 30 years. The results showed that a person's chances of becoming obese increased by 57 percent if she or he had a friend who became obese, by 40 percent if she or he had a sibling who became obese, and by 37 percent if her or his spouse became obese. The infectious effect was greater among friends of the same sex. A 71 percent increased risk of obesity was seen if a same-sex friend became obese (Christakis 2007).

In addition, a person's chances of becoming obese were influenced by his or her family and friends, even if they were hundreds of miles away. How could this possibly occur? The dramatic effect of distant friends on the odds of increased obesity rules out exposure to the same environment as a cause. The Christakis study analyses revealed that similar weights were not due to any tendency for people to interact with others like them, eating the same foods as their friends did, or participating in the same physical activities as their friends did. It may be that esteem for friends influences a person's conception of a normal, healthy, and attractive body size. The investigators found that thinness also appeared to be socially contagious. When a person lost weight and was no longer obese, her or his friends and family tended to lose weight, too. The scientists proposed that this contagious social influence should be exploited to spread positive health behaviors from one person to the entire social network.

Another remarkable theory about how obesity may occur has been put forth by a group of researchers who have implicated a virus in the development of obesity in animals and possibly in humans. In 1992, Nikhil Dhurandhar, at the University of Bombay, reported that an avian adenovirus (Ad36) caused excessive fat in chickens (Dhurandhar 2000). Researchers began to look for antibodies against this type of virus in obese humans. The presence of antibodies against the virus means that the person had been exposed to the virus at some time. When Richard Atkinson, professor of medicine and nutrition at the

University of Wisconsin, Madison, and Dhurandhar screened humans in India and the United States for Ad36 antibodies, they found that approximately 30 percent of the people with obesity had the antibodies, compared with only 10 percent of normal-weight people (Atkinson 2005). The researchers theorize that the virus somehow affects the brain centers that control appetite.

Treatment of Obesity

There are no simple solutions to the obesity problem. Obesity is a complex condition that requires complex solutions. Successful treatment of obesity and overweight requires lifelong behavioral changes rather than short-term weight loss or quick fixes. Programs that emphasize realistic goals, gradual progress, sensible eating, and exercise are recommended by weight loss experts. Those that promise instant weight loss or feature severely restricted diets are not effective in the long run. Unfortunately, the success rate for even sensible diets is approximately 3–5 percent. Studies show that most people regain a considerable amount of weight by one year and nearly everyone returns to her or his pre-diet weight after five (Sumithran 2013).

Long-term management of obesity is the most challenging aspect of weight control for many individuals. Whatever method of weight loss is used, the preferred goals of treatment are similar. In the past, physicians and other experts who designed treatment programs encouraged people to achieve their ideal weight based on height-weight charts or recommended BMI. Given the lack of success in preventing weight regain, most programs now aim for the "10 percent solution"—to lose about 10 percent of body weight. The focus is on improving overall health, rather than attaining a certain weight.

Attempting to lose weight is a common pursuit for many Americans. A study published in 2005 reported that 46 percent of U.S. women and 33 percent of U.S. men said they were trying to lose weight (Bish 2005). The approaches that most people use typically include a combination of dieting, increasing physical activity, lifestyle modification, and behavioral changes. Some dieters try dietary supplements or medications that theoretically could increase or speed up weight loss. For individuals who have not had success with diet, lifestyle, and medication, various types of surgery may be an option.

For those who enjoy a structure of companionship and support while trying to manage weight, a wide variety of weight loss groups are available. Do-it-yourself programs include groups like Overeaters Anonymous (OA) and Take Off Pounds Sensibly (TOPS). These self-help groups are free of charge and are led by group members. TOPS advises a low-calorie, low-fat meal plan, while OA encourages members to abstain from refined foods that might act as triggers to overeat. The OA philosophy helps to guide participants to physical, emotional, and spiritual recovery. Minimal scientific evidence is available to examine success rates from these two groups.

Commercial franchises, like Weight Watchers, Jenny Craig, and Nutrisystem, offer meetings, materials, and even meals. These groups rely on counselors to provide services to clients. In an evaluation of the success of the best-known commercial programs, people who followed the Weight Watchers plan maintained a greater than 5 percent weight loss over 12 months. Participants attending the most group sessions kept off the most weight, clearly showing the importance of staying with the program (Tsai 2005). A 2015 review of 11 popular diet programs revealed that Weight Watchers and Jenny Craig scored highest for effectiveness. However, many other plans were not studied enough to evaluate long-term results.

Most participants remained overweight, with weight loss of between 3 and 5 percent of their initial weight. Even that amount of sustained weight loss may produce healthful benefits, including lower blood pressure and blood glucose (Gudzune 2015).

Clinical programs provided by medical professionals who may have specialized training to treat obese patients focus on

medical nutrition therapy, exercise, and psychological counseling. They can feature very-low-calorie diets (VLCDs) and
liquid diets, medications, and surgery. Medically supervised
proprietary programs, such as Optifast, Health Maintenance
Resources, and Medifast, place patients on very-low-calorie,
high-protein plans (usually about 800 calories per day). These
programs customarily use liquid diets in place of solid food,
and participants are closely monitored by a physician. The theory is that a VLCD could be effective for obese individuals to
start their weight loss, if they have the medical supervision critical for following it safely. Afterward, a transitional period with
measured meal replacements, slow reintroduction to foods, and
education about new ways of healthy eating should help ensure
long-term success. Studies show that patients completing these
programs can lose approximately 15–25 percent of their initial weight during 3–6 months of treatment and maintain a
loss of 8–9 percent at one year (Tsai 2005). The success rate
might be overestimated, as the results did not include those
who dropped out of programs. A task force from the National
Heart, Lung and Blood Institute (NHLBI) has indicated that
one year after the diet is completed, VLCDs do not result in
any greater weight reduction when compared with other, less
stringent diets providing 1,200–1,500 calories (NHLBI 1998).

Several commercial Internet-based programs offer meal
plans, recipes, online chats with other dieters, and e-mail advice from experts such as dietitians and psychologists. Published evidence of outcomes from eDiets showed participants
losing 1.1 percent of their initial weight after one year. This
type of information and support could be used on its own or
could supplement other programs. The convenience of online
record keeping of daily intake and activity could possibly increase weight maintenance.

The struggle to lose unwanted pounds requires choosing
between responsible products and programs that offer methods for achieving moderate weight loss over time and "miracle" products or services that promise fast and easy weight loss

without sacrifice. Advertisements for weight loss products and services flood the marketplace with promises of instant success without the need to give up favorite foods or increase physical activity. An example of such an eye-grabbling ad reads, "Amazing New Discovery, Guarantees Weight-Loss, Eliminates Dieting. . .And Can Slash Up To 29 Pounds Of Embarrassing Fat From Your Body Almost Overnight—Without Wasting 1 Minute Of your Day!" as seen on the Internet at "get-slim-while-you-sleep.com". Almost all weight loss experts agree that the key to long-term weight management requires permanent lifestyle changes that include a healthful diet at a moderate calorie level and regular physical exercise. A large gap remains between recommended dietary patterns and what Americans actually eat. One study reported that 7 out of 10 Americans consume less than the recommended servings of vegetables each day and 25 percent had no daily vegetable intake at all (Casagrande 2007).

With dozens of new diets and miraculous foods being advertised, people find it hard to know what to eat, what to avoid, and whom to believe. For a healthy diet beneficial both for weight loss and for improving long-term health, the U.S. Department of Agriculture's (USDA) *Dietary Guidelines for Americans* provides practical examples of healthful diet choices for everyone. Every five years, HHS and USDA jointly publish the *Dietary Guidelines for Americans* based on the latest scientific evidence. The latest version, in 2015, encourages individuals to focus on foods and beverages that help achieve and maintain a healthy weight, promote health, and prevent chronic disease (USDA 2015). The guidelines are based on the most current authoritative advice about healthful dietary habits and are the basis for federal food and nutrition education programs and are depicted graphically as MyPlate (USDA 2014). MyPlate is based on five food groups—fruits, vegetables, grains, protein foods, and dairy—to incorporate into a healthy plate at meal times. The guidelines are not specifically weight loss diets. They are presented across a range of calorie levels for people over two years of age with recommended calorie intake and food patterns for individuals based on age, sex, and activity level. "USDA Estimated Calorie Needs per Day by Age, Gender, and Physical Activity Level" is a chart that shows the appropriate calories needed for males and females by age and activity level. "USDA Food Patterns" identifies suggested amounts of food to consume from the various food groups at 12 different calorie levels (see Table 5.5 and Table 5.6 in Chapter 5). The entire set of recommendations is intended to be used in the context of planning an overall healthful diet.

However, following *any* of the recommendations can have health benefits. The advice contained in these guidelines related to choosing a variety of healthy foods in correct portions is a good way to maintain a healthy weight. Professional weight management experts generally use the USDA guidelines in combination with other general strategies to reduce calorie intake. Suggestions for personal weight management often include the following advice:

- Make an individualized plan and assessment: Begin with an evaluation of what you are eating. This is called a current diet assessment. The word "diet" brings to mind meals of tuna and carrot sticks or dry toast. A diet is actually all the food and beverages that a person takes in during the course of a day. People generally underestimate how much they eat and often do not remember what they ate from one day to the next; so, keeping a journal that lists actual amounts of all food and beverages consumed can be an effective tool to identify foods that contribute to weight gain (Table 5.7 in Chapter 5). http://ebooks.abc-clio.com/reader.aspx?isbn=9781598841961&id=OBESC-1680—OBESC-1680 is an example of a form for keeping a record of when one eats, what, and how much one is eating, and the hunger level experienced. Using the program entails matching the foods on the form with daily goals in "MyPlate Calorie Levels" and "MyPlate Food Intake Patterns" or using MyPlate

SuperTracker to assess the quality of one's diet. MyPlate SuperTracker is an online, interactive dietary and physical activity assessment tool that translates the principles of the *Dietary Guidelines for Americans* into individualized healthful choices. Personalized recommendations are made for food and activity depending on one's age, sex, and weight. Using this tool helps to point out links between good nutrition and regular physical activity and assists in keeping track of the food and exercise history for up to one year (USDA 2014).

- Reduce energy intake: A 500–1,000-calorie-per-day deficit can theoretically result in a weight loss of 1–2 pounds of fat per week. This type of energy reduction is designed to achieve slow, progressive weight loss, and for most people this means that the reduced energy plan will total about 1,000–1,200 calories for women and 1,200–1,600 calories for men. The MyPlate online tools provide a good guide to meal plans for these calorie levels. Even with some guidelines, evaluating calorie content of foods takes practice because energy content is not always obvious. For a woman with a goal of 1,200 calories per day, just six chocolate sandwich cookies provide more than one-quarter of those calories. Calorie content of foods can be estimated using online databases, food labels, restaurant nutrition information sheets, and handbooks of nutrient information.

- Recognize fat as a concentrated source of energy: Fat is a concentrated source of calories. It has 9 calories per gram, whereas protein and carbohydrate have only 4 calories per gram. Thus, fat can supply more than twice as many calories in each bite as a bite of carbohydrate or protein. In a given weight of food, the most efficient way to reduce calories is to cut back on the fat. In the campaign to prevent obesity, the NHLBI suggested limiting total fat to 30 percent or less of total calories. For example, in a 2,000-calorie diet, about 660 calories—or about 75 grams of fat—could come from fat in meals each day. Historically, studies have shown that people consume more total energy with high-fat diets compared with low-fat diets (NHLBI 1998). However, a 2014 year-long study found that total energy intake was similar between groups whether the diet was low fat or high fat (Bazzano 2014).

- Eat less fat and sugar and more fruits and vegetables: Calorie density of menu items can be diluted by the addition of fruits, vegetables, whole grains, and water. For example, extra vegetables and whole grain bread can reduce the calorie density of a meat sandwich. Plant fiber adds volume and provides a feeling of fullness, so fewer overall calories may be consumed.

- Limit food quantity at home and when eating out: By recalibrating portion sizes to fit individual health goals, it is possible to eat all types of foods in moderation at home or when eating out. Even without measuring spoons or cups, the amount of a standard food portion may be visualized by comparison to objects of similar size. For example, three ounces of meat or poultry is about the size of a deck of cards or the palm of one's hand. One-half cup of cooked rice, pasta, or potato is similar in size to half of a baseball or the amount that can fit in a cupped hand. A serving size card with more examples of what one serving looks like can be downloaded at http://hp2010.nhlbihin.net/portion/keep.htm.

Dozens of complex diets have been promoted for weight loss, but there is no scientific evidence to show that any one diet is more effective than another. Table 5.8 in Chapter 5 helps sort through the various types of diets that exist today. It lists some of the most common diet plans, examines their advantages and disadvantages, and provides the dietary basis behind their potential benefits.

There is considerable interest in the effects of individual macronutrients—fat, protein, and carbohydrate—to make weight management easier or more effective. High-carbohydrate, high-fiber, low-fat diets, like those proposed by Dean Ornish and Nathan Pritikin, include whole grains, fruits, and vegetables. These diets limit all types of dietary fat. Fat is not intrinsically bad, but because fat contains twice the calories of protein or carbohydrate, reduced fat meals provide more food volume for fewer calories.

High-fat, high-protein, low-carbohydrate food plans, such as the Atkins diet, may be more satisfying than low-fat diets. With this approach, it is possible that less food would be eaten, but weight loss does not occur unless fewer calories are consumed overall. A review of nearly 100 studies of low-carbohydrate weight loss diets did not find enough evidence to recommend for or against the use of such diets. Weight loss was related to eating fewer calories and staying on the diet for a longer period of time, but not with the carbohydrate content of food (Bravata 2003). At this time, no reliable data are available to show that any combination or avoidance of foods will work better than the others over the long term. The closer a person follows any calorie-reduced diet, the greater the weight loss. It is the adherence to a diet and not the diet itself that makes the difference (Thomas 2014; http://ebooks.abc-clio.com/reader.aspx?isbn=9781598841961&id=OBESC-743 — OBESC-926).

Another widely held opinion about dieting, even among health professionals, is that weight lost rapidly is more quickly regained. Gradual weight loss is recommended. To test the effect of the rate of weight loss on the rate of regain in obese people, an Australian trial randomly assigned 200 participants to gradual weight loss or rapid weight loss programs. At the end of the study, both gradual and rapid weight loss participants had regained most of their lost weight (gradual weight loss 71% regain vs rapid weight loss 70% regain). The rate of weight loss had no significant effect on weight maintenance (Purcell 2014). No one intervention works equally for everyone. Not everybody loses weight. Of those who do so, the majority are unable to keep it off. Before experts are able to predict that diet plans will actually cause weight loss for longer than six months, they need more data about matching the diet intervention to individual metabolic and social needs.

Diet Foods

The U.S. food and beverage industries have launched massive campaigns to develop and promote reduced calorie foods using products such as artificial sweeteners and fat replacers. It is not certain how these foods contribute to weight management for most Americans. Do people actually lose weight by snacking on fat-free chips and sugar-free puddings? Perhaps, they just feel free to eat more of everything. Although it seems to make sense that exchanging high-calorie sweeteners with sugar-free substitutes could help control weight, no scientific consensus has been reached regarding their value. A study, in which participants were given either water or diet drinks, showed that the no-calorie beverage group lost significantly more weight compared to the water group (13 vs. 9 pounds) after 12 weeks. Participants in the diet drinks group also reported feeling less hungry than those in the water group (Peters 2014). Other randomized, controlled trials involving these sweeteners have generally shown only that they produced only modest weight loss (Brown 2012). It was suggested that they could only be a benefit if they are integrated into a reduced-calorie diet (Fitch 2012). Although some investigators have concluded that artificial sweeteners enhance weight loss, others have suggested that they actually increase body weight. This idea is based on studies such as one in France that showed that people who regularly consume artificial sweeteners have a higher BMI (West 2001). Instead of suggesting a causal relationship between artificial sweeteners and increased body weight, these data may reflect practices in which individuals were using artificial sweeteners to reduce calories because they were already overweight. Little is known about the long-term impact of sweetener replacements on energy intake and body weight.

The American Heart Association and the American Dietetic Association report that fat substitutes can have a substantial impact on weight reduction as long as they lower total calorie intake (Wylie-Rosett 2002). Olestra, which goes by the brand name Olean, is a synthetic mixture of sugar and vegetable oil that passes through the body undigested. It was approved for use as a replacement for fats and oils in prepackaged ready-to-eat snacks by the FDA in 1996. Olestra-based foods have the sensory qualities of real fat; however, concern has been expressed about its safety based on reports from individuals who experienced gastrointestinal problems, such as cramps and loose stools, after consuming large amounts of olestra. Olestra has lost its popularity due to side effects, but products containing the ingredient can still be found in some grocery stores.

Several studies on the effects of olestra on appetite and energy intake showed that replacement of dietary fat with olestra resulted in weight loss that was significantly greater than a control diet. In these studies, weight loss occurred because total energy intake was reduced. The overall results from studies of sugar and fat replacers and increased dietary fiber indicate that some products used to reduce energy density are helpful in obesity management, while others do not make a significant contribution. The essential factor that determines effectiveness of modified food products is that total calories in a person's meals and snacks must be decreased, or the benefit of energy-reduced foods for weight management is limited (Bray 2004).

Nutritionists caution the public to be aware of the realities of the modest weight reduction potential of reduced calorie foods. The realities are that calories do count (Kazaks 2008). Calories consumed must equal calories expended even with low-energy-density foods. A reduced calorie food label is not a license to eat unlimited amounts guilt free. Low-calorie products should be used as substitutes for higher calorie foods, not in addition to a regular diet. Furthermore, lower calorie foods should taste good. Not all products provide desirable flavors, aromas, and textures. The promises of successful weight management by reduced calorie food consumption is based on the theory that following a reduced calorie diet is easier when the taste and qualities of sugars and fats are provided in reduced calorie versions of foods. It is anticipated that the volume of food in low-calorie, high-fiber products may help consumers be satisfied with smaller portions at each meal and, consequently, fewer calories overall.

Adequate Nutrition Labeling

Nutrition labels can help consumers make the informed food choices that contribute to a healthy diet. In 1990, the Nutrition Labeling and Education Act (NLEA) was signed into law. This act was a new mandate for food manufacturers to disclose the fat (saturated and unsaturated), cholesterol, sodium, sugar, fiber, protein, and carbohydrate content in their products. It required retailers to provide labels for their store's 20 top-selling fruits, vegetables, fish, and shellfish, although meat, poultry and egg products, infant formula, foods sold in bulk, foods with insignificant amounts of nutrients, and foods sold by retailers with total sales of less than $500,000 were exempt from the requirement. Retailers did not have to label each item, but if they chose not to, they were required to provide this information in a single location in the store.

In 1993, the FDA and the USDA issued regulations that specified the table format and content of nutrition labels on most foods, including processed meat and poultry products. The nutrition facts table is intended to contain easy-to-read and easy-to-use information that allows purchasers to understand the nutritional value of a food, compare products, and increase or decrease consumption of nutrients or calories. More details related to the Nutrition Facts Label may be found in the Resources Chapter.

Although consumers have the right to nutrition information about food products, NLEA did not cover foods purchased in restaurants and at prepared food counters in grocery stores. Despite the fact that people are eating more food away from home, usually they can only guess at the calorie content of the items they order. Most restaurants have no trouble listing the price of menu items, but only about a third provide nutrition information on the menus. Without having the information right where the food purchasing decision is made, most people have difficulty comparing options and making the most healthful choice. A study conducted in 2006, with more than 5,000 Americans who answered questionnaires about their food purchases, revealed that, on average, they ate away from home about six times per week. In that study, consumers agreed that they were ultimately responsible for making sensible food choices; however, 41 percent wanted to see more nutrition information printed on menus so they could choose well (Mallone 2005). The Institute of Medicine, FDA, Office of the Surgeon General, and AMA all called for prominently visible displays of calories and other nutrition information at the point of choice in restaurant chains. The Center for Science in the Public Interest, a consumer advocate group whose goals are to counter the food industry's influence on public opinion and public policies and to lobby for government policies, was at the forefront of efforts to make calorie content of purchased food readily available.

In 2006, the New York City Department of Health and Mental Hygiene became the first agency to require most restaurants to show calorie information on menus and menu boards. In 2007, the New York State Restaurant Association (NYSRA) challenged the regulation and it was subsequently blocked. The Department of Health loosened some of the rules that the NYSRA had objected to and reinstated the menu-labeling regulation. A subsequent motion filed by chain restaurant lobbyists to again block the requirement that the calorie value of dishes must be displayed alongside prices was rejected by a U.S. District Court judge. The judge agreed with the argument that showing calorie values alongside prices will help consumers make choices that will lead to a lower incidence of obesity, and the regulation went into effect in 2008. The judge's ruling meant that any restaurant chain with 15 or more nationwide outlets, or about 10 percent of the restaurants, in the boroughs of New York City—Manhattan, Brooklyn, Queens, the Bronx, and Staten Island—were required to display calorie counts on menus, menu display boards, and food tags. Advocates of menu labeling say this landmark decision paved the way for other local and state governments to pass similar measures.

Early in 2014, 20 years after the first standardized label regulations took effect, the FDA announced that it would update the Nutrition Facts Labels to display calorie counts more prominently and to include the amount of added sugars (FDA 2014a). Later that year, the FDA went even further, announcing new rules that required chain restaurants and vending machine operators to post calories for food and drinks on their menus and machines. The policies, which had been proposed as part of the 2010 Affordable Care Act (ACA), apply to restaurants that have more than 20 locations nationwide. The rules also include labeling requirements for restaurant-style food in grocery stores, big-box stores, coffee shops, ice cream stores, movie theaters, and amusement parks. The concepts behind the creation of the new food labels were to better inform the public about what they are consuming, while encouraging industry to create healthier products (FDA 2014b).

Physical Activity

As discussed previously, moderate exercise does not greatly contribute to weight reduction. Exercise does use up calories, and the cumulative effects of regular exercise over long periods of time can be beneficial in preventing weight gain. However, calorie expenditure from low-level activity is not adequate to permit increased food intake. When individuals have unrealistic expectations that exercise can increase weight loss, they may become disappointed at the lack of results. The true benefits of exercise are preventing weight gain, decreasing body fat, maintaining weight loss, and improving general health at any weight. For long-term good health, an important goal is to establish a regular, sustained pattern of physical activity (Wadden 2000).

Behavioral Strategies for Responding to an Obesogenic Environment

Living in an obesogenic environment—one that encourages sedentary living and aggressively promotes consumption of high-energy-density foods—requires increasing effort to overcome this barrier to good health. Behavioral treatment of overweight and obesity trains individuals to gain control over unhealthful external conditions, as they identify and modify personal dietary and physical activity responses that lead to overweight. Four behavioral strategies commonly applied to weight loss and maintenance programs are (1) self-monitoring, (2) stimulus control, (3) cognitive restructuring, and (4) social support (Fujioka 2002).

Self-monitoring diet and exercise patterns: To change behaviors, it helps people to become aware of their actions such as overeating or being sedentary. Keeping a journal listing all food and beverages consumed and the duration and frequency of physical activity can be an effective learning tool because it pinpoints the amounts and types of food eaten and exercise performed each day. Daily food and activity records provide immediate feedback, so a problem pattern becomes obvious and possible solutions can be tried right away. Self-monitoring data can be recorded in a diary or notebook, as entries into a handheld computer, or with the use of a computerized diet and exercise analysis program. Exercise can be monitored in time or distance, as with the use of a pedometer. People generally underestimate how much they eat and overreport exercise. Record keeping decreases the tendency of both lean and obese people to underestimate their food intake (Kretsch 1999). Reducing energy intake is the key to weight reduction, and accurate assessment of food intake by keeping food records is consistently related to weight loss (NHLBI 1998).

Stimulus control: Personal diet and activity records can identify the "triggers," or environmental cues associated with incidental eating, overeating, and inactivity. Generally, weight-management guides, diet books, and Web sites provide a wide variety of tips or ideas for managing cues.

Cognitive restructuring—defining weight loss success: If dieters are to develop reasonable weight loss goals, they must correct false beliefs and expectations. Most dieters have unrealistic ideas about the amount of weight they want to lose and the extent of weight loss that is possible with even the best treatment. Instead of aiming for ideal weight based on the Metropolitan Life Insurance Company's height-weight charts, people should target a 10 percent reduction in body weight, as suggested earlier, for a successful outcome. Losing as little as 5–10 percent of initial weight has been shown to improve hypertension, type 2 diabetes, and abnormal cholesterol levels, even if the person is not at ideal body weight (NHLBI 1998). Most individuals expect that dieting will result in much more weight lost than these modest goals. A study, published in 2000, reported that participants who lost 10 percent of their body weight during a four-month treatment were disappointed and felt that they had failed because their weight loss was not, to them, sufficient (Foster 2001). In this study, nearly 400 women beginning a weight loss program were asked to describe their goal weight loss in terms of what they wished to achieve, what they would be happy with, and weight loss they would view as unsuccessful. The women said they aimed for about a 38 percent reduction in body weight—more than three times the recommended goal. A 25 percent reduction was described as just "acceptable," but not one they would be happy with. A 16 percent loss was considered "disappointing." These responses suggest that many dieters have unrealistic goals and, even after a medically significant weight loss, they may feel unsuccessful. Cognitive restructuring is also useful in dealing with lapses or weight regain. Individuals are encouraged to see the setback for what it is—a temporary lapse from which it is possible to recover, instead of total failure. The setback is assessed to determine why the lapse occurred and how a similar situation could be prevented in the future. Other techniques include rehearsing ways to cope with relapse before it occurs. Each time a challenge is successfully managed—even an imaginary one—the chances of relapse are reduced (Wadden 2000).

Social support network: People with a social support network are more successful at weight loss and maintenance than those without strong support systems. Sixty-six percent of women who participated in behavior modification groups along with friends were able to maintain total weight loss 10 months after treatment compared with only 24 percent of those in the group of people who were recruited alone (Wing 1999). Scientific literature on weight maintenance of greater than three years shows that diet combined with group therapy and social support have the best chance of long-term success (Ayyad 2000). Most weight is lost during the first six months of treatment (Wadden 2000). Numerous studies show that weight loss is enhanced by long-term behavioral treatment, but attendance at sessions generally declines over time, and without support and encouragement and having to be accountable for healthful lifestyle choices, people regain weight. For most dieters, about a third of the initial weight loss is regained in the year after treatment. Three to five years later, at least 50 percent of participants have returned to their initial weight or gained more. Behavioral maintenance therapy can delay weight regain, but data are insufficient to prove that it is effective over the long term (Kramer 1989).

Long-Term Success

The National Weight Control Registry (NWCR) shows that some people are successful at long-term weight management on their own. The NWCR was a project developed in 1994 by Dr. Rena Wing and Dr. James Hill to help identify those individuals who have succeeded at long-term weight maintenance and to examine the strategies that were successful. An estimated 5,000 people participate in the NWCR. Participants may register if they have maintained at least a 30-pound weight loss for more than a year. After studying these individuals, Hill and colleagues first described the keys to their weight loss success in a 2005 article. In essence, no one plan or diet was common to all participants. Weight loss was maintained by a variety of personally designed diet and exercise strategies. Many participants had tried and failed several times before they were able to find the lifestyle and diet patterns that worked for them. Methods that were common to most participants were eating a relatively low-fat diet, eating breakfast, self-monitoring through food records, weighing themselves regularly, and regular physical activity (about one hour per day; Hill 2005). A follow-up 2014 study of NWCR participants, who had kept lost weight off for 10 years, showed that larger initial weight losses were associated with better long-term outcomes. Decreases in leisure time physical activity and increases in percentage of energy intake from fat were associated with greater weight regain. The researchers reported that the majority of weight lost by NWCR members is maintained over 10 years. Long-term weight loss maintenance is possible; however, it requires long-lasting behavior change (Thomas 2014). At present, no strategies are defined that will help the majority of obese and overweight people successfully manage their weight, given an environment that encourages overeating and less and less physical activity. Because millions of people are overweight or obese, they are a diverse group and it is possible to take many routes to success.

Medications: Nonprescription

Numerous over-the-counter (OTC) weight loss products are available; most have not been proven to be effective and safe. During the past decades, products for weight loss have been required to change their formulations based on updated government regulations and warnings. For example, amphetamines, originally developed as a treatment for narcolepsy, were introduced in 1937 as weight loss drugs when they were found to reduce appetite as well as keep people awake. An amphetamine-type drug, desoxyephedrine, was approved by the FDA for obesity treatment in 1947.

Amphetamines

In 1960, amphetamines were the most commonly prescribed medications for obesity (Parry 1973). Amphetamines were not without risks. Accelerated heart rate, increased blood pressure, hallucinations, psychiatric disorders, addiction, withdrawal problems, and heart failure were side effects that brought about the end of the amphetamine era. In the 1970s, government agencies all over the world placed tighter restrictions on drugs with the potential for abuse. Stimulant drugs are well established in treatment of obesity, and amphetamines are still approved for use under tight regulations in most countries.

Ephedra

Ephedra, also commonly known as Ma Huang, has been used in Chinese medicine for more than 2,500 years. It is made of dried branches of an evergreen shrub-like plant native to Central Asia and Mongolia. The principal active ingredient, ephedrine, is a compound that can powerfully stimulate the nervous system and heart. Ephedrine is chemically similar to amphetamines and may decrease appetite and increase metabolism. From the 1980s, ephedra had been popular for increasing energy and enhancing athletic performance, and it was used in many dietary supplements marketed for weight loss, but legal issues concerning its health risks went back and forth. It was banned in the United States by the FDA in 2004 because of safety concerns. In 2005, the ban was overturned by a federal District Court judge in Utah in response to a suit brought by an ephedra manufacturer. The FDA appealed this lower court ruling, and in 2006 the U.S. Court of Appeals for the Tenth Circuit upheld the original ban. With 19,000 adverse events reported, it was concluded that no dose of ephedrine was safe and the sale of these products in the United States was made illegal. Up until this ruling, many supplement companies marketed low-dose ephedra products containing 10 milligrams (mg) or less of ephedra. According to the FDA, there is little evidence to show that ephedra is effective except for short-term weight loss. Any benefits are outweighed by increased risks of hypertension, heart attacks, strokes, or seizures (NCCAM 2013).

Another drug, phenylpropanolamine, originally used to treat nasal congestion, also had the side effect of appetite suppression and was used in nonprescription diet aids for weight loss. One such product was Dexatrim—a popular diet pill for more than 25 years. Phenylpropanolamine was Dexatrim's primary ingredient, but it was removed from the product line because of side effects such as increased risk for bleeding in the brain. Dexatrim switched its focus to ephedrine-based pills until ephedrine was banned by the FDA. After the ban, manufacturers of diet and weight loss drugs, like Dexatrim, turned their attention to finding alternatives that would mimic its effects. Dexatrim products are now drug free. They are based on a blend of guarana, kola nut, and bitter orange as well as several vitamins and minerals; green tea extract is also a common ingredient. They may or may not contain caffeine. Some side effects may include dizziness, nausea, high blood pressure, and depression. Dexatrim does point out that its diet aid works best when used with a sensible meal plan and regular exercise. It advertises that dieters will see results in one to two weeks when diet, exercise, and Dexatrim diet pills are combined. The truth is that most people could probably achieve the same results with diet and exercise alone.

The Metabolife line is another group of popular OTC products. Metabolife 356, an ephedra-based supplement, once generated hundreds of millions of dollars in annual sales. Metabolife 356, like other ephedra-containing supplements, was linked to thousands of serious adverse events; so, it was discontinued following the FDA ban on ephedra-containing dietary supplements. Currently, Metabolife offers various supplements for weight loss or weight maintenance phases that may contain caffeine; vitamins; minerals; and caffeine-containing extracts of green tea, guarana, and yerba mate. Even without the effective ephedra, the plan still claims that the supplement will control appetite and burn fat. Metabolife also recommends that its products be combined with a healthy diet and exercise program. To support that advice, an online program helps consumers plan and track weight loss goals through education, tips from the experts, and community encouragement. The Web site features a collection of healthy recipes; suggestions for strength-training exercises, weight management tips, and logs to track goals, diet, fitness, and results. Using Metabolife without changes in lifestyle will not be helpful for weight loss because it does not contain ingredients that have been proven to achieve effective results in the long run. The FDA does not support the weight loss promises made by Metabolife.

For people who are wondering whether any OTC weight loss medications work, the answer is, maybe. Although some ingredients like caffeine or tea that increase energy expenditure may be helpful for weight control, the concentration of these ingredients in diet preparations probably is too small to have an effect on weight loss in most people. A few cups of coffee or tea could have a similar outcome, taste better, and cost much less.

Herbs and Supplements

A popular question among people who are looking for more ways to control weight is: "What herbs or supplements should I take to lose weight?" A survey indicated that more than a quarter of American women trying to lose weight tried OTC weight loss supplements (Blanck 2001). The products promise a wide variety of ways to reduce fat, including increasing energy expenditure, increasing satiety, increasing fat oxidation, and blocking dietary fat and carbohydrate absorption. In terms of OTC weight loss products, 64 percent of consumers think the government requires warnings about potential side effects, 54 percent believe these products are approved for safety by the FDA, and 46 percent think the products are approved for efficacy. In addition, 37 percent of consumers believe that herbal supplements are safer than prescription or OTC medications (Pillitteri 2008). None of these beliefs is true. Although claims that dietary supplements can prevent, mitigate, treat, or cure a specific disease cannot be legally made, this distinction becomes clouded for many weight loss products. Misleading weight loss claims are seemingly everywhere, preying on consumers desperate for an easy solution. Current regulatory processes are weak, underfunded, and understaffed.

Supplements are attractive because they often advertise remarkable benefits and they are marketed as "natural," which may be interpreted as an assurance of safety and efficacy. The choice to supplement a diet with particular botanicals, vitamins, minerals, or other products can be a sensible decision that improves well-being and vitality. How do we sift through the false claims or junk science to find accurate information about supplements and their side effects or benefits? Because there is no official recommended dose for supplements, distributors are free to say whatever they want to about products. Intriguing research findings may be seen in animals; however, rats and mice are not people. Clinical trials with humans are necessary to know if the supplements are truly effective. Only carefully controlled scientific studies can show whether a product actually works. The best information is based on the results of rigorous scientific testing, rather than on testimonials or anecdotes. Some supplement suppliers accuse scientists of trying to keep secrets about alternative products that have miraculous powers. However, scientists are interested in studying the benefits and the risks of dietary supplements. The federal government even has an agency, the National Center for Complementary and Integrative Health (NCCIH), devoted to rigorous scientific research on complementary health products and practices. Anyone can get information on thousands of studies from the NCCIH website.

Example of Research Study in Detail: Chitosan Dietary Fiber Supplement

Fiber supplements and "fat blockers" have been advertised as ways to prevent fat absorption and produce weight loss. Following is an example of research that shows how scientists assessed the claims and effectiveness of chitosan, a fiber supplement, starting with some background on the product.

Chitosan is a calorie-free, high-fiber carbohydrate. It is produced commercially by chemically altering chitin, which is the structural element in the shells of crustaceans such as crabs, shrimp, and lobsters. As a food ingredient, chitosan adds thickness and a smooth texture to food products and is used in applications such as thickening chocolate milk drinks. Chitosan also has been approved by the FDA for use as an edible film to protect foods from dehydration. Like other forms of fiber, such as bran, chitosan is not well digested by the human body. Chitosan's configuration allows it to bind to fats and cholesterol. Its calorie-reducing effect is ascribed to its purported ability to bind with ingested fat and carry it out of the digestive tract. It has been used in Japan in several types of foods, including soybean paste, potato chips, and noodles, to help prevent fat absorption. A Japanese confection called Choco Lady is a sweet chocolate pellet that contains a crispy chitosan-enriched center. The pellets are claimed to help with weight loss. The product description states: "For maximum effect, the consumer is advised to eat five pellets before each meal. . .targeted towards men and women who tend to eat greasy meals" (AFJ 2006).

Apart from its role as a food additive, chitosan is sold as a dietary supplement with claims that it will block the absorption of significant amounts of dietary fat and lead to rapid weight loss. In support of the fat-blocking claim was a demonstration aired on the QVC television channel. A beaker was filled with oil and a water-based liquid to simulate what happens in a person's gastrointestinal tract, even though a beaker does not actually simulate human digestion. When the oil and water did not mix, chitosan was added to the concoction. The TV camera showed clumps of chitosan. This demonstration is offered as "proof" that chitosan combines with fat, prevents it from being absorbed by the body, and will lead to rapid weight loss. If chitosan were to work as claimed, an increased amount of fat would appear in the feces after a person consumes chitosan along with meals containing fat. A series of studies that measured the amount of fat in feces of a total of 104 men and women taking chitosan were published in 2005 (Gades 2005). These data were compared with data from a control period. Three different brands of chitosan were tested. The greatest amount of fat that was excreted in men was 1.8 grams per day, or 16 calories. At that rate, it would take more than 15 months to lose about 2 pounds of body fat using chitosan. It did not block the absorption of any fat in women. A systematic review of randomized controlled trials of chitosan indicated that the effect of chitosan on body weight was minimal and unlikely to be of clinical significance (Mhurchu 2005).

Red Flag Campaign

The allure of a magic elixir can tempt anyone who wants an easy way to lose weight. Consumers spend roughly $1 billion a year on heavily advertised weight loss products that are at best unproven and at worst unsafe. They promote unrealistic expectations and false hopes. In September 2002, the U.S. Federal Trade Commission (FTC) released a report titled *Weight Loss Advertising: An Analysis of Current Trends* indicating that the use of false and misleading claims in weight loss advertising was widespread (FTC 2002). Researchers examined 300 weight loss advertisements taken from television, radio, the Internet, newspapers, magazines, e-mail, and direct mail. The Commission found that 55 percent of weight loss ads made claims that were misleading, lacked proof, or were obviously false. Although the FTC study did not criticize specific products, it provided numerous examples of false or exaggerated claims and said some weight loss supplements lacked safety warnings and could be dangerous.

The FTC Division of Advertising Practices is responsible for enforcing federal truth-in-advertising laws. In 2014, the Division published *Gut Check: A Reference Guide for Media on Spotting False Weight Loss Claims* that includes a list of seven advertising claims that are likely to be a tip-off to deception. If a product contains any of these claims, the FTC suggests that advertisers think twice before running any ad that says a product:

1. causes weight loss of two pounds or more a week for a month or more without dieting or exercise;
2. causes substantial weight loss no matter what or how much the consumer eats;
3. causes permanent weight loss even after the consumer stops using product;
4. blocks the absorption of fat or calories to enable consumers to lose substantial weight;
5. safely enables consumers to lose more than three pounds per week for more than four weeks;
6. causes substantial weight loss for all users; or
7. causes substantial weight loss by wearing a product on the body or rubbing it into the skin (FTC 2014).

Prescription Medications: History and Current Weight Loss Options

Fen-Phen

In 1992, a University of Rochester professor first promoted the drug combination of fenfluramine and phentermine, or fen-phen, as a magic weight loss pill. Studies had shown that the combination could be used in lower dosages with fewer side effects than either drug alone (Weintraub 1984). Participants of a four-year research project lost an average of about 31 pounds on fen-phen versus 10 pounds on a placebo (pill without the drug) after 34 weeks, and they were able to keep the weight off over the long term (Weintraub 1992). The initial rationale for the combination was that the two drugs would provide an additive action, allowing the use of lower, safer doses of each drug. Reviewers from Texas A&M University concluded that the combination was not merely additive but also synergistic—that is, they were more effective together than simply doubling the dose of either drug alone. Mass marketing of this combination of drugs took place, and the number of prescriptions written for fen-phen grew from 60,000 in 1992 to 18 million in 1996 (Langreth 1997). Hundreds of clinics opened specifically to prescribe these weight loss medications. It seemed as though researchers had finally found the magic pill for weight loss and long-term weight control.

The drug was extensively used until a report from the Mayo Clinic linked 24 cases of heart valve disease, which included severe deformity and leakage, to use of the medications. These 24 cases, all women, had no previous history of cardiovascular disease. The leakage was caused by a buildup of abnormal tissue on the valves of their heart that prevented them from sealing properly. This type of valve damage is a silent condition, causing no symptoms until it becomes severe, is life threatening, and requires surgery to repair. Another investigation showed that 271 of 291 patients who had taken fen-phen showed abnormal electrocardiograms. In 1997, American Home Products, fen-phen's manufacturer, removed the drug from the market (Langreth 1997). The 50-year-old generic drug phentermine, which was one-half of the fen-phen combination, does not show these serious side effects and is still on the market.

Meridia

Meridia was FDA-approved in 1997 as a long-term appetite suppressant. Meridia is the brand name for sibutramine, a selective serotonin reuptake inhibitor. The drug prevents recycling (re-uptake) of noradrenaline and serotonin. Noradrenaline and serotonin are neurotransmitters that enhance the feeling of satisfaction from eating. Weight loss with sibutramine is increased when positive changes are made in diet and lifestyle. In one trial, people with an initial BMI of 30–40 who had lost weight when given sibutramine for four weeks continued to lose weight during 44 additional weeks of sibutramine treatment.

In this study, people were simply told to eat a healthy diet. However, in another study, a much higher amount of weight loss was achieved when sibutramine treatment was combined with lifestyle modification counseling. Those who had sibutramine alone lost an average of 11 pounds after a year, while those in the sibutramine plus counseling group had an average weight loss of 26 pounds (Rubio 2007).

The neurotransmitters that control appetite also control numerous other body processes, so side effects from sibutramine are common. The drug was not recommended for people with hypertension because it increased blood pressure in some individuals. Other reported side effects include constipation, dry mouth, headache, and increased heart rate. Meridia was also associated with more serious problems. Between February 1998 and September 2001, hundreds of people throughout the world who took Meridia were hospitalized, and the FDA reported that 29 people taking Meridia in the United States had died.

In 2002, sibutramine encountered regulatory problems. Warnings about its safety had been issued in France and the United Kingdom. The Italian Ministry of Health suspended sales of the drug after 50 reports of adverse events and two deaths. However, the European Union Committee for Proprietary Medicinal Products later issued a report stating that, when used according to directions, sibutramine had a favorable risk/benefit ratio. The manufacturer, Abbott Laboratories, had reported that the death rate among patients taking the drug (12,000 people in clinical trials and 8.5 million patients worldwide) was substantially lower than what would normally occur in any obese patient population (Abbott 2002). In the United States, the FDA conducted an investigation into the safety of the drug, and in 2010 Meridia was voluntarily withdrawn from the United States and Canadian markets. Data from a post-marketing study, the Sibutramine Cardiovascular Outcomes Trial, indicated that individuals with cardiovascular disease had an increased risk of heart attack and stroke with this drug (James 2010).

Orlistat

Hoffmann–La Roche's Xenical is the brand name for orlistat, an obesity drug that can be taken for an extended time period. It blocks fat-digesting enzymes in the intestine called lipases and prevents some dietary fat from being digested and absorbed. It is usually taken three times a day before main meals that contain fat. Up to 30 percent absorption of dietary fat can be blocked with 120 mg of orlistat taken with a meal. This extra fat that passes down the intestine may cause abdominal pain, gas, oily stools, and fecal incontinence, especially if the fat content of the meal is high. This effect persuades users to limit their fat intake.

A meta-analysis of Xenical trials showed that the drug helped dieting patients lose an average of 2–3 percent of their body weight compared with dieting alone. After one year of treatment, about one-third more patients treated with orlistat three times per day lost a greater percentage of body weight than those treated with placebo. In a number of studies, orlistat treatment significantly improved blood pressure, lowered levels of LDL cholesterol (bad cholesterol) in the blood, and lowered fasting blood glucose and insulin levels. Results from a four-year study suggested that development of type 2 diabetes, especially in those with impaired glucose tolerance, was delayed with orlistat use (Heymsfield 2000). The majority of subjects across the studies gained the weight back after discontinuing the drug.

Orlistat has been approved for OTC sales as the product Alli. It contains about half the dose of the prescription drug. The package insert cautions that, while the product does prevent fat absorption, it may cause oily bowel movements so frequently that it suggests consumers wear a panty liner when starting the treatment.

Rimonabant

Rimonabant, a drug marketed by Sanofi-Aventis, acts, both in the brain and in other parts of the body, to increase feelings of fullness, and it plays a role in the metabolism of glucose and fat. It is an inhibitor of cannabinoid type 1 receptors, which are widely distributed in the brain and in other tissues, including on fat cells. Interestingly, these receptors affect intake of sweet or fatty foods. These same receptors are also involved in nicotine addiction; thus, rimonabant is also prescribed to help people quit smoking. Overeaters and smokers have been shown to have very active cannabinoid type 1 receptors. In clinical trials in people with BMI values of 34–38, participants taking rimonabant had a significantly greater weight loss after one year compared with those given a placebo. By continuing rimonabant treatment for a second year, weight loss was maintained. Subjects who were switched to a placebo regained most of the weight they had lost in the first year (Rubio 2007). Rimonabant was authorized for use in Europe and other countries, but never approved in the United States because an FDA advisory panel unanimously recommended against approving the drug because of its side effects, including risk of depression and suicide. The drug was withdrawn from the global market in 2009 and it is no longer under development.

Response to drug therapy varies among individuals and no one drug works for all people. Diet drugs will not force anyone to stop eating, as most people eat in response to environmental cues rather than physiologic hunger. Medical professionals are beginning to understand that regain of weight upon stopping medication is not treatment failure, but rather it indicates that obesity is a chronic disease much like diabetes. Drugs are not a quick fix for a disease that requires long-term treatment. It would be helpful to have weight loss medications that can be used for long periods of time, such as those used for treatment of hypertension and dyslipidemia. As risks are inherent in taking any medication, research is needed to assess the long-term safety of obesity drugs relative to the health risks of obesity and overweight.

In 2012, the FDA approved two drugs for long-term weight loss: lorcaserin hydrochloride (Belviq; Eisai Inc.) and phentermine-topiramate (Qysmia; Vivus Inc.).

They were the first drugs to be approved in over a decade since orlistat was allowed in 1997. Lorcaserin is thought to promote weight loss by targeting receptors in the brain that generate a sense of satiety. Phentermine-topiramate is a combination drug: phentermine is a sympathomimetic agent that suppresses appetite, and topiramate is an antiepileptic drug that was noted to cause weight loss as a side effect (Woloshin 2014). Given the health risks of previous weight loss drugs, it makes sense to ask, "How effective and safe are these medications?" The approvals were based on 1-year trials showing that, in addition to recommendations to follow a calorie-restricted diet and to increase exercise, patients randomized to either drug lost more weight than patients randomized to a placebo (3% more weight lost with lorcaserin and 7% more with phentermine-topiramate). To judge weight loss drugs, the FDA considers two criteria: Do people lose 5 percent or more of their body weight with the drug versus placebo? Do at least 35 percent of people taking the drug lose at least 5 percent of their body weight (and the percentage lost in the treatment group is at least double the percentage lost in the placebo group)? Lorcaserin met one of these criteria; phentermine-topiramate met both (Woloshin 2014). Drug therapy and lifestyle interventions are not opposing strategies; it is recommended that the current drugs used for weight loss are combined with lifestyle interventions. Neither medication was marketed in Europe because of safety concerns. The drugs' labels include warnings about memory, attention, or language problems and depression and cardiovascular abnormalities.

Obesity (Bariatric) Surgery

In 1954, Dr. Arnold Kremen and Dr. John Linner at the University of Minnesota were studying nutrition absorption in dogs. They discovered that the dogs lost weight after they underwent operations that bypassed much of their intestines (Kremen 1954). After Dr. Linner went into private surgical practice, one of his patients asked him to use the technique on her in the hope that she, too, could lose weight. With the successful results of that procedure, bariatric surgery was born. In 1991, an NIH expert panel endorsed bypass surgery for obesity when they reviewed what was known about surgical treatments for severely overweight individuals. It concluded that surgical alterations of the digestive system appeared to work for many people without severe side effects. It approved bariatric surgery as an effective option for severely obese people who have failed more moderate weight reduction strategies. In 1999, singer Carnie Wilson had gastric bypass surgery and allowed the procedure to be broadcast live over the Internet. The broadcast was viewed by more than 500,000 people. Sixteen months after the procedure, Carnie had lost 152 pounds of her original weight of more than 300 pounds. She was a celebrated example of successful weight loss surgery, and even posed for *Playboy Magazine* in 2003. In 2005, after she gave birth to her daughter, the pounds began to come back. In 2008, she weighed more than 200 pounds—her weight had increased but still down about 100 pounds from her heaviest. Wilson tried again to lose weight when she received laparoscopic band surgery in 2012. That the weight may be eventually regained demonstrates a limitation of obesity surgery. On the other hand, an important health benefit is that the procedure may allow individuals to gain many years of reduced risk related to high levels of obesity.

Official guidelines consider weight loss surgery appropriate for adults with severe obesity (BMI $\geq$ 40, or 37–39.9, if accompanied by other conditions such as diabetes) who have not reached a satisfactory weight through diet, exercise, and medication. Surgery may be used as the initial treatment if BMI is greater than or equal to 50. It is major surgery, undertaken only by specialist hospital teams, and is not without risks. People who have weight loss surgery will need continuing specialist medical support for many years. Weight loss surgery is not advised in children, except in extreme circumstances.

Some types of weight loss surgery that are currently used are gastric banding, sleeve gastrectomy, and gastric bypass. In gastric banding, a small pouch is made in the upper part of the stomach with an adjustable band and the main part of the digestive system is unchanged. In this purely restrictive procedure, the new smaller pouch fills up quickly, produces a sensation of fullness, and reduces food intake. The food passes slowly into the main part of the stomach, and then on to the rest of the digestive system. The surgery is most often done with laparoscopy; therefore, it is called laparoscopic adjustable gastric banding. In laparoscopic surgery, both a small video camera and surgical instruments are inserted through small incisions made in the abdomen allowing the surgeon to conduct and view the procedure on a video monitor. A remarkable feature of the gastric band is that it can be adjusted without additional surgery. The band is actually a balloon filled with saline solution that can be inflated or deflated. This operation causes weight loss by reducing food intake, leaves the main part of the digestive system unchanged, and is reversible. It typically produces a 40–50 percent loss of excess body weight in the two years after surgery (FDA 2014c).

Another technique is called a "sleeve gastrectomy." During this procedure, about 75 percent of the stomach is removed leaving a narrow tube or "sleeve". The new, smaller stomach is about the size of a banana. No intestines are removed or bypassed during the sleeve gastrectomy. It limits the amount of food one can eat and increases the feeling of fullness after eating just small amounts of food. It is not simply a mechanical reduction effect, since the cells that manufacture hunger hormones, such as ghrelin, also are removed resulting in a decreased appetite in people who have this surgery.

In the gastric bypass procedure, the top section of the stomach is partitioned to make a new mini stomach. This pouch is connected to a lower section of the small intestine, bypassing the upper part where most active digestion takes place. Food does not get broken down normally in the smaller stomach, and absorption of nutrients from the small intestine is greatly reduced. Weight loss is caused by both restriction and reduced absorption of food. The surgery results in about 55–65 percent of excess body weight (WIN 2011).

Obesity Surgery Benefits and Cautions

Pros

Following obesity surgery, most patients experience rapid weight loss and continue to do so for 12–18 months. Some patients may maintain 50–60 percent of their weight loss 10–14 years after obesity surgery.

Cons

Several risks are associated with obesity surgery, including a 10 percent or higher risk of complications. It is estimated that 10–20 percent of patients may need follow-up operations to correct obesity surgery complications such as abdominal hernias. Gallstones develop in more than one-third of patients. Anemia, osteoporosis, and other bone diseases are the result of nutritional deficiencies that develop after the obesity surgery. The possible death rate, 1 out of 200 cases, is lower for more experienced surgeons who perform at least 150 operations yearly (Morino 2007). Blue Cross and Blue Shield of North Carolina's assessment of results of surgery for morbid obesity showed that success rates were highly variable in their coverage area. Some surgeons had significant complication rates of 25–50 percent. By reviewing the claims data, the company found that patients of physicians who performed bariatric procedures more often had lower complication rates. Complications included such events as gastrointestinal tract leakage, bowel obstruction, bleeding, infections, complications from anesthesia, and death. With the expectation that the complication rate should be less than 10 percent during the first 60 days, Blue Cross identified those programs that consistently delivered high-quality results as Bariatric Surgery Centers of Excellence (Pratt 2006).

Despite much progress in developing safer and more effective surgical techniques, obesity surgery remains a last option for patients attempting weight loss. In addition, surgical candidates must be willing to radically change the way they eat to reflect the very much smaller amount of food (and water) that can be consumed at one time. One of the side effects of this surgery is the decreased absorption of some vitamins. Patients take a pre-scribed multivitamin pill that has larger doses of vitamins than the standard multivitamin supplement. The surgery commonly allows patients to reduce 50 percent of their *excess* weight. A person who is 100 pounds overweight could theoretically maintain a 50-pound loss and be healthier but still overweight. Long-term weight loss is not effortless after bariatric surgery. Lifestyle change is still necessary. For many people, the stomach pouch enlarges, intestinal absorption increases, and weight can be regained if diet and physical activity are not changed also.

Other Invasive Treatments for Obesity

Jaw Wiring

In 1977, the concept of wiring the jaws together was intro-duced. Jaw wiring can be performed in a dentist's chair; it is a painless procedure that takes less than an hour to perform. This orthodontic method of weight control prevents consumption of solid food, thus causing a reduction in calorie intake. Once the desired weight loss is achieved, the wiring is removed. The success rate of jaw wiring as a long-term method to achieve a normal weight is very low. Most patients do not discover a new, healthful way of eating; in fact, some are able to sip enough high-calorie fluids through a straw that no weight is lost at all. Large clinical studies demonstrated a median weight loss of 55 pounds with jaw wiring, but after four months the weight loss reached a plateau. When the wires were removed, patients re-gained 100 percent of the lost weight (Farquhar 1986).

Liposuction

Liposuction is the most popular form of cosmetic surgery. It is a surgical procedure that removes fat deposits from areas under the skin (abdomen, thighs, buttocks, neck, back of arms) that do not respond to traditional weight loss methods. The fat is extracted with a vacuum suction cannula (a hollow pen-like instrument) or with an ultrasonic probe that breaks up the fat, and then removes it with suction. The cosmetic effect of liposuction may be very good, and many patients report being satisfied. Liposuction is not a cure for obesity, because relatively little body fat (less than 10 pounds) can be removed safely. Some side effects include unusual lumpiness or dents in the skin, excessive bleeding, and negative response to general or local anesthesia. Because fat removal is considered a cosmetic procedure, most medical insurance will not pay for liposuction. The fat that is removed may come back with weight gain. Furthermore, the fat may appear in areas of the body where it did not previously occur (FDA 2014d).

How Does the Health Care System Deal with Obesity?

The health care system has a responsibility to play an active role in the management of obesity, and physicians are a first line of defense in addressing the issue. A major barrier to successful weight management is the lack of communication between patients and their health care providers. Despite the current focus on obesity and health care risks, less than half of obese patients are advised by their physicians to lose weight. Seventy-five percent of patients surveyed indicated that they looked to their physician a "slight amount" or "not at all" for help with weight control (Wadden 2000). When physicians mention weight, they often do not give useful, actionable information. Because patients have trouble losing weight and maintaining weight loss, they need ongoing support and reinforcement from health care providers. In an interview with Dr. William Dietz, obesity and nutrition expert from the Centers for Disease Control and Prevention, he said:

The kind of care delivery system necessary for chronic diseases like obesity is different from the traditional patient-provider relationship. So many patients in the

United States are overweight that the one-to-one provider-patient relationship is probably archaic. It is based on an acute care model whereby the U.S. medical system has evolved to treat infectious diseases or injuries. It did not evolve to treat chronic diseases, and it did not evolve around prevention. Providers are not financially rewarded when they prevent disease; they are rewarded when patients get sick or need hospitalization (Pellerin 2005).

Opinion varies widely about how health care providers should manage obesity in the medical office or clinic. Physicians are often reluctant to discuss weight-related issues with patients. Such discussions are time consuming and no solutions are available that apply to everyone, although several studies have shown that physician advice encouraging weight management significantly increases patients' attempts to lose weight (Loureiro 2006). Experts recommend that doctors weigh and measure all their adult patients and refer people with obesity to intensive counseling and behavioral treatment. An individual may want to lose weight but not be ready to make a focused commitment. Health care providers can assess patient willingness to change and educate patients about the effects of overweight on health by discussing results of physical exams, lab tests, and family history. Reduction of excess weight requires concentration and sustained effort. In cases where family or work-related stress interferes with that effort, the treatment goal may simply be prevention of further weight gain (Wadden 2000).

All patients, no matter their weight, can benefit from lifestyle guidance to prevent weight gain. This advice and education will become part of good health care if insurance companies reimburse for obesity management, as they do for control and prevention of diabetes. To deal with the obesity issue, those who are obese or at risk of becoming obese should be offered appropriate long-term interventions, as suggested by the NHLBI guidelines shown in Figure 5.3 in Chapter 5. The algorithm in Figure 5.3 depicts the NHLBI Expert Panel's treatment decision process, which provides a step-by-step approach to managing overweight and obese patients.

Interventions may include individual or group behavior change therapy, pharmaceutical intervention, or surgery for those at highest risk. A crucial step is to provide a variety of programs that can actually help patients manage weight. Because there is no single approach that works for everyone, the most effective interventions offer a number of programs that apply to specific groups. Overall, the most successful strategies rely on an active lifestyle that includes reasonable amounts of healthful foods. While pursuing these health strategies, individuals may need to explore personal associations between emotions and eating habits. Programs may use Web-based resources combined with conventional lifestyle management classes or one-on-one sessions.

With support from health care professionals, self-management is a cornerstone of therapy. Providers cannot be expected to manage weight for their patients. There are no guarantees for any medical treatment, including surgery, for long-term weight loss. The role of the provider is to help patients identify and solve problems that make it difficult for them to maintain a healthy weight. In the end, using the resources currently available, patients must make the choices and manage their problems for themselves.

Why Can't We Just Prevent Obesity?

No one can escape the basic law of nature that governs weight gain or loss—any energy consumed as food and not used through activity must be stored in the body as fat. However, people vary in their eating and exercise habits; in their genetic susceptibility to gaining weight; and in their individual metabolic rate, which determine weight gain or loss. Scientists have discovered a great deal about how weight gain occurs and some methods that may be effective in reversing it, although there is still much to learn. Inability to lose excess weight often has more to do with social, psychological, and behavioral factors than with metabolism. Both physiology and society work against people's weight loss attempts. The automatic slowdown in our metabolic rate with weight loss—an evolutionary protection to prevent starvation—works against us when we try to lose excess weight. Influences of food advertising and the customs of social eating add to the difficulty. In short, weight management is not easy for most people.

Prevention has the potential to help decrease obesity, but no studies have been conducted for a long enough period to indicate what method(s) of prevention will work. Health care professionals and patients continue to question whether they can afford to wait for better evidence. Should we keep trying the methods we now have and hope that they work for some people? The experts' best guesses, given current knowledge, are to encourage people to be more active, reduce marketing of unhealthful foods, and make foods, like fruits and vegetables, more affordable, attractive, and easily available.

Obesity as a Public Health Issue

Public health professionals view those social, economic, and environmental conditions that promote excess weight gain as modifiable factors. Public health leadership to develop and support innovative approaches and partnerships at all levels, from the individual to the community and nation, are needed to address the problem of obesity. Policies such as educational programs to increase physical activity and regulation of advertising of high calorie foods or beverages to children are based on a desire to reduce the problem of obesity, particularly in childhood. Prevention of child obesity, and thereby reducing future risk of obesity in adulthood, is one of the most important public health issues facing the nation (Macdonald 2011). In 2010, Surgeon General Regina Benjamin, emphasized prevention in her message: *A Vision for a Healthy and Fit Nation.* Dr. Benjamin's directive was for a change in focus from a negative one about obesity and after-the-fact medical treatments to a positive one aimed at prevention and being healthy and fit. She outlined opportunities obesity prevention interventions involving personal behaviors and biological traits, and also on the social and physical environments that encourage or limit opportunities for positive health outcomes (Benjamin 2010).

An examination of public health strategies reveals how the focus has changed over the last decade. Prior to 2008, the national approach to obesity focused on personal responsibility and providing education about the dangers of obesity and how each person could improve health habits. After 2008, the federal government initiated a number of new or revised obesity-related programs targeted to environments such as schools, worksites, health care organizations, and communities as well as individual behaviors.

As an example, in 2011, the CDC released *School Health Guidelines to Promote Healthy Eating and Physical Activity* (NCHS 2011) to provide science-based guidance for schools on establishing a school environment supportive of healthy eating and physical activity. The report included up-to-date scientific evidence and current best practices as it also incorporated the 2010 *Dietary Guidelines for Americans*, the 2008 *Physical Activity Guidelines for Americans*, and the objectives for *Healthy People 2020*. See the Data and Documents chapter for more details about obesity and school health guidelines.

The *Dietary Guidelines for Americans* encourage individuals to eat a healthful diet that focuses on foods and beverages that help achieve and maintain a healthy weight, promote health, and prevent chronic disease. The guidelines are updated every five years by the HHS and the USDA. A Dietary Guidelines Advisory Committee, consisting of nationally recognized experts in the field of nutrition and health reviews current scientific and medical knowledge, provides a report for the next edition of the *Guidelines*. The advisory report is not the definitive *Guidelines* policy. First, the public gets an opportunity to view the report and provide written comments, and then the HHS and USDA use all the information to develop and release the new *Guidelines* (ODPHP 2015).

In 2008, the first-ever *Physical Activity Guidelines for Americans* were developed by the Office of Disease Prevention and Health Promotion (ODPHP) within HHS. These *Guidelines* are needed because of the importance of physical activity to the health of Americans, whose current inactivity puts them at unnecessary risk. The guidelines aim to reduce the proportion of adults who engage in no leisure time physical activity at all, and to increase the proportion of adolescents and adults who actually do meet current guidelines (HHS 2009).

The *Healthy People* initiative provides science-based national goals and objectives designed to guide national health promotion and disease prevention efforts within the 10-year targets (HHS 2011). The current *Healthy People 2020* is based on evaluation of the accomplishments and deficiencies of four previous decades of *Healthy People* programs.

Because coordination is essential among government agencies and other sectors in society, leadership at the national level is vital to move the obesity and health agenda forward. In 2010, First Lady Michelle Obama assumed such leadership when she launched the Let's Move! program with the ambitious goal of eliminating childhood obesity within a generation. The First Lady brought together public officials, the food industry, advocacy groups, and others to raise public awareness about the impact of environmental aspects of obesity. A Let's Move! Web site was created to offer tips and tools for how to raise healthy children at home and in schools. A link to the Web site is in the Resources section. As part of this coordination effort, President Barack Obama established the Task Force on Childhood Obesity to identify key benchmarks and outline a national action plan. The Task Force Report presented a series of recommendations structured around the same four goals of the First Lady's Let's Move! initiative: (1) empower parents and caregivers to make healthy choices for their families; (2) serve healthier food in schools; (3) ensure access to healthy, affordable food; and (4) increase physical activity (Letsmove.org 2010).

Affordable Care Act and Labeling

The year 2010 also brought the ACA, which expanded benefits and coverage of services for obesity prevention. An important provision was new nutrition labeling requirements. The ACA required chain restaurants with 20 or more locations to post calorie and nutrition information on menus, menu boards, drive-through displays, and certain vending machines. The FDA was charged with regulating and detailing how the law would be carried out. Readily available nutrition information on menus and menu boards is thought to be a great benefit for weight management since well-informed consumers can make healthier choices. In a report from the Yale Rudd Center for Food Policy and Obesity, 80 percent of consumers said they wanted calorie information (Rudd 2011). Leading health organizations, including the AMA, agree that nutrient labeling that is easy to understand is necessary. Several states and localities had already led the way by enacting menu labeling laws before the ACA requirements.

At that time, and currently, it is not yet clear what effect calorie labeling has on food choices and obesity. In 2009, researchers examined the influence of required menu labeling on fast food choices in New York City where nearly 1,200 adults who ate at fast food restaurants were compared with a sample in Newark, New Jersey, which had no menu labeling law. More than a quarter of the New York City diners said the calorie information influenced their food choices. However, when researchers analyzed what diners actually bought, there was no difference in the number of calories purchased by the two groups (Elbel 2009). In a study, investigators examined consumers' behavior at Starbuck's coffee stores and determined that the average number of calories per transaction fell by 6 percent when calories were prominently posted. Researchers found that in areas where menu labeling is mandatory, restaurants were

58 percent more likely to offer low-calorie options than restaurants in other areas (Bollinger 2010).

Industry

It is not just government agencies that are responsible for nationwide obesity management strategies. Every segment of society plays an important part in reducing obesity. Industries that shape food availability and physical activity environments should be recognized as partners that can respond to public and private concerns about nutrition and obesity while still meeting their business need to turn a profit (Huang 2009). The Partnership for a Healthier America (PHA), an independent, nonpartisan organization, was created in 2010 with a mandate to mobilize the private sector, foundations, media, and local communities to action around the goals of the Let's Move! campaign. The PHA committed to bringing healthy, affordable food to nearly 10 million people with new stores in low-income areas that lacked opportunities to purchase affordable and nutritious foods close to home. First Lady Michelle Obama declared, "We can give people all the information and advice in the world about healthy eating and exercise, but if parents can't buy the food they need to prepare those meals because their only options for groceries are the gas station or the local minimart, then all that is just talk" (The White House 2011).

In the summer of 2011, Wal-Mart and McDonald's reported that they planned to make major changes in the way they marketed their products. Wal-Mart announced that it would open 300 stores in areas without access to fresh produce and healthy foods. McDonald's reformulated its children's Happy Meals to contain apple slices and 1.1 ounces of fries, instead of the original 2.4 ounces of fries without any fruit. McDonald's made changes to its menu by adding new salads, oatmeal, and smaller portions of dessert in an effort to position itself as a healthier fast food chain.

In cooperation with the PHA, the Healthy Weight Commitment Foundation (HWCF), a food industry-led organization, voluntarily pledged to make healthful foods more available in the marketplace (HWCF 2010). The coalition includes hundreds of retailers, food and beverage manufacturers, restaurants, sporting goods companies, insurance companies, trade associations, nongovernmental organizations, and professional sports organizations. The Robert Wood Johnson Foundation (RWJF), a founding PHA member, was responsible for conducting a rigorous, independent evaluation of HWCF efforts to provide healthful foods to American consumers and to publicly report the findings (Lavizzo-Mourey 2009). The companies, acting together as part of the HWCF, had pledged to remove 1 trillion calories from the marketplace by 2012 and 1.5 trillion by 2015. This reduction would bring the calories available in the marketplace to what they were in 2008. The Foundation members pursued calorie reduction in several ways:

- Product reformulation and innovation;
- Offering smaller portions;
- Redesigning packaging and labeling;
- Placing calorie information on the front of products;
- Providing consumers with information and educational materials;
- In-store promotion of the HWCF initiative (HWCF 2010).

The real challenge of creating new calorie-reduced products is that they must also satisfy consumer expectations for convenience, taste, quality, and price.

In 2013, the RWJF evaluation found that the companies sold 6.4 trillion fewer calories in the United States in 2012 than they did in 2007, and had exceeded their 2015 goal by more than 400 percent (Ng 2014). Investigators found that the largest calorie reductions in HWCF brands were in fats/oils, soft drinks, ready-to-eat cereals, and candy. This evidence seems to indicate a great benefit for reducing obesity in the United States, but some public health advocates question the actual value of simple calorie reduction. There were no increases seen in sales of HWCF brand foods linked to weight loss and lower risk of cardiovascular diseases, such as fruits, nuts/seeds, vegetables, seafood, and yogurt. In addition, during the same time period, annual calories sold by non-HWCF brands rose by 1.4 trillion (Mozaffarian 2014).

Strategic Plan for NIH Obesity Research

Potentially successful models for obesity prevention encompass dietary, activity, behavioral, pharmacological, and surgical components targeted to individual needs. To answer the questions and controversies surrounding obesity prevention and treatment, scientific research into lifestyle or medical approaches that will make it easier for anyone to maintain a healthful energy balance is necessary. People in the United States depend upon the NIH to elucidate the roles of forces that contribute to obesity and to develop strategies for obesity prevention and treatment. The 27 institutes and centers of NIH provide direction and financial support for this effort through competitive grants to researchers in the United States and throughout the world. Currently, the NIH funds more than 90 percent of all obesity research in the United States.

The NIH presented its second Strategic Plan for NIH Obesity Research in 2011. That version updated the first Plan that was released in 2004. The new guide promotes a broad spectrum of obesity research to move science efficiently from laboratory to clinical trials to everyday practice (NIH 2011). Furthermore, research to identify and reduce health disparities underlies all the strategic plan themes. See the Data and Documents chapter for more details about NIH obesity research.

Summary

In an individualistic society, such as the United States, making healthy choices is ultimately the responsibility of the individuals and families. However, the larger food culture and environment contributes greatly to the weight problems that are so prevalent in the population. The public health challenge is to acknowledge and build upon individual responsibility beliefs to generate personal and collective responsibility approaches in ways that will help reduce the incidence of overweight and obesity. It is important that local and national policy is shaped to help people make choices for a healthful lifestyle by removing obstacles and by creating more opportunities to be healthy. As Marlene Schwartz, deputy director for the Rudd Center for Food Policy and Obesity at Yale University asserts, "It's great for people to be responsible, but we have to make it easy for them. We have to create an environment that facilitates responsibility" (Hobson 2009).

Researchers, experts, and government policy makers have suggested ways to change the food and activity environment to provide healthier options in communities, schools, and worksites. Many of these tactics are particularly aimed at underserved groups of people whose options have been most limited. Proponents of using taxes and laws to improve access to a healthful food and activity environment for everyone point to other government-directed public health successes. The theory is that if taxes and laws can get Americans to wear seat belts and to stop smoking, they can also persuade the general population to exercise more and eat better. The food industry and industries that shape the built environment are also responsible for creating an environment that will keep their customers healthy. Because consumers are becoming more interested in the benefits of nutritious foods and physical activity, creative and astute industry leaders can market and advertise attractive and healthful products that are part of a profitable business model.

New initiatives, such as the Surgeon General's Vision for a Healthy and Fit Nation 2010, Let's Move!, the ACA, and other federal policy changes, have provided new opportunities to support antiobesity efforts. Developing and initiating these programs is important, but that is only the first step. These policies must be fully implemented and funded. However, tough economic climates create obstacles, particularly major cuts to federal, state, and local governments. When governments at all levels face difficult budget decisions, it is critical to think about both sides of the ledger: cuts to obesity programs today could mean higher health costs and a less healthy workforce later (Levi 2011). The basic message from evaluations of previous and continuing programs and interventions is that reversing the obesity epidemic will be a long-term effort. It will require individuals, families, schools, communities, businesses, government, and other organizations to work together and to use new research to find effective ways to apply obesity-related science to practical, realistic applications.

References

Abbott. Abbott Laboratories. 2002. Accessed January 6, 2009. http://www.meridia-rx.com/diet-pills/meridia/meridia_safety.htm.

AFJ. "Choco Lady (Japan)." 2006. *Asian Food Journal.* Accessed January 6, 2009. http://www.asiafoodjournal.com/print.asp?id=3580.

Atkinson, R. L., N. V. Dhurandhar, D. B. Allison, R. L. Bowen, B. A. Israel, J. B. Albu, and A. S. Augustus. "Human Adenovirus-36 is Associated with Increased Body Weight and Paradoxical Reduction of Serum Lipids." *International Journal of Obesity* 29, no. 3 (2005): 281–286.

Ayyad, C., and T. Andersen. "Long-Term Efficacy of Dietary Treatment of Obesity: A Systematic Review of Studies Published between 1931 and 1999." *Obesity Reviews* 1, no. 2 (2000): 113–119.

Bazzano, L. A., T. Hu, K. Reynolds, L. Yao, C. Bunol, Y. Liu, C. S. Chen, M. J. Klag, P. K. Whelton, and J. He. "Effects of Low-Carbohydrate and Low-Fat Diets: A Randomized Trial." *Annals of Internal Medicine* 161, no. 5 (2014): 309–318.

Benjamin, R. *The Surgeon General's Vision for a Healthy and Fit Nation 2010.* Rockville, MD: Office of the Surgeon General Department of Health and Human Services, 2010.

Bish, C. L., H. M. Blanck, M. K. Serdula, M. Marcus, H. W. Kohl, 3rd, and L. K. Khan. "Diet and Physical Activity Behaviors among Americans Trying to Lose Weight: 2000 Behavioral Risk Factor Surveillance System." *Obesity Research* 13, no. 3 (2005): 596–607.

Blanck, H. M., L. K. Khan, and M. K. Serdula. "Use of Nonprescription Weight Loss Products: Results from a Multistate Survey." *The Journal of the American Medical Association* 286, no. 8 (2001): 930–935.

Bravata, D. M., L. Sanders, J. Huang, H. M. Krumholz, I. Olkin, and C. D. Gardner. "Efficacy and Safety of Low-Carbohydrate Diets: A Systematic Review." *The Journal of the American Medical Association* 289, no. 14 (2003): 1837–1850.

Bray, G. A., S. Paeratakul, and B. M. Popkin. "Dietary Fat and Obesity: A Review of Animal, Clinical and Epidemiological Studies." *Physiology and Behavior* 83, no. 4 (2004): 549–555.

Breymaier, S. "AMA Adopts New Policies on Second Day of Voting at Annual Meeting." 2013. American Medical Association. Accessed December 8, 2014. http://www.ama-assn.org/ama/pub/news/news/2013/2013–06–18-new-ama-policies-annual-meeting.page.

Brown, R. J., and K. I. Rother. "Non-Nutritive Sweeteners and Their Role in the Gastrointestinal Tract." *The Journal of Clinical Endocrinology and Metabolism* 97, no. 8 (2012): 2597–2605.

Carmona, R. *The Obesity Crisis in America.* Edited by Surgeon General U.S. Public Health Service. Washington, DC: Department of Health and Human Services, 2003.

Casagrande, S. S., Y. Wang, C. Anderson, and T. L. Gary. "Have Americans Increased Their Fruit and Vegetable Intake? The Trends between 1988 and 2002." *The American Journal of Preventive Medicine* 32, no. 4 (2007): 257–263.

Center for Consumer Freedom (CFF). *Epidemic of Obesity Myths*. Washington, DC: Center for Consumer Freedom, 2004.

Christakis, N. A., and J. H. Fowler. "The Spread of Obesity in a Large Social Network over 32 Years." *The New England Journal of Medicine* 357, no. 4 (2007): 370–379.

Dea, F. "A Promising Milestone in Coverage for Obesity Treatments." 2014. The Obesity Society. Accessed December 8, 2014. http://www.obesity. org/publications/a-promising-milestone-in-coverage -for-obesity-treatments.htm.

Dhurandhar, N. V., B. A. Israel, J. M. Kolesar, G. F. Mayhew, M. E. Cook, and R. L. Atkinson. "Increased Adiposity in Animals Due to a Human Virus." *The International Journal of Obesity and Related Metabolic Disorders* 24, no. 8 (2000): 989–996.

Elbel, B., R. Kersh, V. L. Brescoll, and L. B. Dixon. "Calorie Labeling and Food Choices: A First Look at the Effects on Low-Income People in New York City." *Health Affairs (Millwood)* 28, no. 6 (2009): w1110–w1121.

Ernsberger, P. "Obesity Is Hazardous to Your Health: Negative." In *Debates in Medicine* 2. 9th Revision, edited by Gary Gitnick, 102–37. St. Louis, MO: Mosby, 1989.

Farquhar, D. L., J. M. Griffiths, J. F. Munro, and F. Stevenson. "Unexpected Weight Regain Following Successful Jaw Wiring." *Scottish Medical Journal* 31, no. 3 (1986)): 180.

FDA. "Proposed Changes to the Nutrition Facts Label." 2014a. U.S. Food and Drug Administration. Accessed December 18, 2014.

http://www.fda.gov/Food/GuidanceRegulation/
GuidanceDocumentsRegulatoryInformation/
LabelingNutrition/ucm385663.htm.

FDA. "Menu and Vending Machines Labeling Requirements."
2014b. U.S. Food and Drug Administration.
Accessed January 15, 2015. http://www.fda.gov/Food/
IngredientsPackagingLabeling/LabelingNutrition/
ucm217762.htm.

FDA. "Gastric Banding." 2014c. U.S. Food and Drug
Administration. Accessed December 10, 2014. http://www.
fda.gov/MedicalDevices/ProductsandMedicalProcedures/
ObesityDevices/ucm350132.htm.

FDA. "Liposuction Information." 2014d. U.S. Food
and Drug Administration. Accessed December 10,
2014. http://www.fda.gov/MedicalDevices/
ProductsandMedicalProcedures/SurgeryandLifeSupport/
Liposuction/default.htm.

Federal Trade Commission (FTC). "Weight-Loss Advertising:
An Analysis of Current Trends." 2002. U.S. Federal Trade
Commission. Accessed December 10, 2014. https://www
.ftc.gov/reports/weight-loss-advertisingan-analysis-current-
trends.

Federal Trade Commission (FTC). "Gut Check: A Reference
Guide for Media on Spotting False Weight Loss Claims."
2014. U.S. Federal Trade Commission. Accessed
December 10, 2014. http://www.business.ftc.gov/do
cuments/0492-gut-check-reference-guide-media-spo
tting-false-weight-loss-claims.

Fitch, C., and K. S. Keim. "Position of the Academy of
Nutrition and Dietetics: Use of Nutritive and Nonnutritive
Sweeteners." *The Journal of the Academy of Nutrition and
Dietetics* 112, no. 5 (2012): 739–758.

Flegal, K. M., B. I. Graubard, D. F. Williamson, and M. H.
Gail. "Excess Deaths Associated with Underweight,

Overweight, and Obesity." *The Journal of the American Medical Association* 293, no. 15 (2005): 1861–1867.

Foster, G. D., T. A. Wadden, S. Phelan, D. B. Sarwer, and R. S. Sanderson. "Obese Patients' Perceptions of Treatment Outcomes and the Factors That Influence Them." *Archives of Internal Medicine* 161, no. 17 (2001): 2133–2139.

Fujioka, K. "Management of Obesity as a Chronic Disease: Nonpharmacologic, Pharmacologic, and Surgical Options." *Obesity Research* 10, no. 2, Suppl. (2002): 116S–123S.

Gades, M. D., and J. S. Stern. "Chitosan Supplementation and Fat Absorption in Men and Women." *Journal of the American Dietetic Association* 105, no. 1 (2005): 72–77. Accessed August 15, 2007. http://www.ncbi.nlm.nih.gov/pubmed/15635349.

Gregg, E. W., Y. J. Cheng, B. L. Cadwell, G. Imperatore, D. E. Williams, K. M. Flegal, K. M. Narayan, and D. F. Williamson. "Secular Trends in Cardiovascular Disease Risk Factors According to Body Mass Index in US Adults." *The Journal of the American Medical Association* 293, no. 15 (2005): 1868–1874.

Gudzune, K. A., R. S. Doshi, A. K. Mehta, Z. W. Chaudhry, D. K. Jacobs, R. M. Vakil, C. J. Lee, S. N. Bleich, and J. M. Clark. "Efficacy of Commercial Weight-Loss Programs: An Updated Systematic Review." *Annals of Internal Medicine* 162, no. 7 (2015): 501–512.

Healthy Weight Commitment Foundation (HWCF). "Fact Sheet Healthy Weight Commitment Foundation Initiative to Reduce Calories in the Marketplace." 2010. Accessed August 15, 2011. http://www.healthyweightcommit.org/news_media/media_resources/.

Heymsfield, S. B., K. R. Segal, J. Hauptman, C. P. Lucas, M. N. Boldrin, A. Rissanen, J. P. Wilding, and L. Sjostrom. "Effects of Weight Loss with Orlistat on Glucose Tolerance and Progression to Type 2 Diabetes in Obese

Adults." *Archives of Internal Medicine* 160, no. 9 (2000): 1321–1326.

Hill, J. O., H. Wyatt, S. Phelan, and R. Wing. "The National Weight Control Registry: Is It Useful in Helping Deal with Our Obesity Epidemic?" *The Journal of Nutrition Education and Behavior* 37, no. 4 (2005): 206–210.

Hobson, Katherine. "If Diets Don't Work, What's the Solution to Obesity in America?" 2009. *US News & World Report* (March 5). Accessed August 1, 2011. http://health. usnews.com/health-news/managing-your-healthcare/ diabetes/articles/2009/03/05/if-diets-dont-work-whats-th e-solution-to-obesity-in-america.

Huang, T. T., A. Drewnosksi, S. Kumanyika, and T. A. Glass. "A Systems-Oriented Multilevel Framework for Addressing Obesity in the 21st Century." *Preventing Chronic Disease* 6, no. 3 (2009): A82.

Internal Revenue Service (IRS). *Internal Revenue Service Ruling 2002–19*. Washington, DC: IRS, 2002.

James, W. P., I. D. Caterson, W. Coutinho, N. Finer, L. F. Van Gaal, A. P. Maggioni, C. Torp-Pedersen, et al. "Effect of Sibutramine on Cardiovascular Outcomes in Overweight and Obese Subjects." *The New England Journal of Medicine* 363, no. 10 (2010): 905–17.

Kazaks, A., and J. S. Stern. "Strategies to Reduce Calories in Foods." In *Handbook of Obesity, Clinical Applications*, edited by G. A. Bray and C. Bouchard, 417–424. New York: Informa Healthcare, 2008.

Kochanek, K., S. L, Murphy, J. Q Xu, E. Arias. *Mortality in the United States, 2013. Data Brief, no 178*. Hyattsville, MD, National Center for Health Statistics, 2014.

Kramer, F. M., R. W. Jeffery, J. L. Forster, and M. K. Snell. "Long-Term Follow-Up of Behavioral Treatment for Obesity: Patterns of Weight Regain among Men and Women." *International Journal of Obesity* 13, no. 2 (1989): 123–36.

Kremen, A. J., J. H. Linner, and C. H. Nelson. "An Experimental Evaluation of the Nutritional Importance of Proximal and Distal Small Intestine." *Annals of Surgery* 140, no. 3 (1954): 439–448.

Kretsch, M. J., A. K. Fong, and M. W. Green. "Behavioral and Body Size Correlates of Energy Intake Underreporting by Obese and Normal-Weight Women." *Journal of the American Dietetic Association* 99, no. 3 (1999): 300–306; quiz 307–308.

Kushner, R. F. "Weight Loss Strategies for Treatment of Obesity." *Progress in Cardiovascular Diseases* 56, no. 4 (2014): 465–472.

Langreth, R. "Critics Claim Diet Clinics Misuse Obesity Drugs." *Wall Street Journal*, March 31, 1997.

"Let's Move!" Accessed March 10, 2015. http://www.letsmove.gov.

Levi, J., L. M. Segal, and E. Gadola. *F as in Fat: How Obesity Policies Are Failing in America—2007*. Washington, DC: Trust for America's Health, 2007.

Levi, J., St. R. Laurent, L. M. Segal, and D. Kohn. *F as in Fat 2011: How the Obesity Crisis Threatens America's Future*. Washington, DC: Trust for America's Health, 2011.

Loureiro, M. L., and R. M. Nayga, Jr. "Obesity, Weight Loss, and Physician's Advice." *Social Science and Medicine* 62, no. 10 (2006): 2458–2468.

Macdonald, I. A., and R. Atkinson. "Public Health Initiatives in Obesity Prevention: The Need for Evidence-Based Policy." *International Journal of Obesity* 35, no. 4 (2011): 463.

Mallone, C., and J. Bland-Campbell. "New Insights on the Away-From-Home Eating Patterns and Nutritional Preferences of Americans." 2005. Aramark. Accessed January 9, 2009. http://www.andjrnl.org/article/S0002–8223%2807%2901059–0/abstract.

Mhurchu, C. N., C. Dunshea-Mooij, D. Bennett, and
A. Rodgers. "Effect of Chitosan on Weight Loss in
Overweight and Obese Individuals: A Systematic Review
of Randomized Controlled Trials." *Obesity Reviews* 6, no. 1
(2005): 35–42.

Morino, M., M. Toppino, P. Forestieri, L. Angrisani, M. E.
Allaix, and N. Scopinaro. "Mortality after Bariatric
Surgery: Analysis of 13,871 Morbidly Obese Patients from
a National Registry." *Annals of Surgery* 246, no. 6 (2007):
1002–1007; discussion 1007–1009.

Mozaffarian, D. "The Healthy Weight Commitment
Foundation Trillion Calorie Pledge: Lessons from a
Marketing Ploy?" *The American Journal of Preventive
Medicine* 47, no. 4 (2014): e9–e10.

National Center for Complementary and Alternative
Medicine (NCCAM). "Ephedra." 2013. Accessed
December 8, 2014. https://nccih.nih.gov/health/ephedra.

National Center for Health Statistics (NCHS). *School Health
Guidelines to Promote Healthy Eating and Physical Activity.*
Edited by the National Center for Health Statistics:
Centers for Disease Control and Prevention, 2011.

National Heart, Lung, and Blood Institute (NHLBI). *Clinical
Guidelines on the Identification, Evaluation, and Treatment
of Overweight and Obesity in Adults: Executive Summary.*
Bethesda, MD: National Institutes of Health, 1998.

National Institutes of Health (NIH). *Strategic Plan for
NIH Obesity Research. A Report of the NIH Obesity
Research Task Force NIH.* Edited by National Institutes of
Health: United States Department of Health and Human
Services, 2011.

Ng, S. W., M. M. Slining, and B. M. Popkin. "The Healthy
Weight Commitment Foundation Pledge: Calories Sold
from U.S. Consumer Packaged Goods, 2007–2012." *The
American Journal of Preventive Medicine* 47, no. 4 (2014):
508–519.

Office of Disease Prevention and Health Promotion (ODPHP). "Scientific Report of the 2015 Dietary Guidelines Advisory Committee." 2015. Accessed November 20, 2014. http://www.health.gov/dietaryguideli nes/2015-scientific-report/02-executive-summary.asp.

Parry, H. J., M. B. Balter, G. D. Mellinger, I. H. Cisin, and D. I. Manheimer. "National Patterns of Psychotherapeutic Drug Use." *Archives of General Psychiatry* 28, no. 6 (1973): 18–74.

Pellerin, C. "The Global Epidemic of Obesity." 2005. eJOURNAL USA. Accessed August 18, 2008. http://usa. usembassy.de/etexts/soc/ijge0105.pdf.

Peters, J. C., H. R. Wyatt, G. D. Foster, Z. Pan, A. C. Wojtanowski, S. S. Vander Veur, S. J. Herring, C. Brill, and J. O. Hill. "The Effects of Water and Non-Nutritive Sweetened Beverages on Weight Loss during a 12-Week Weight Loss Treatment Program." *Obesity (Silver Spring)* 22, no. 6 (2014): 1415–1421.

Pillitteri, J. L., S. Shiffman, J. M. Rohay, A. M. Harkins, S. L. Burton, and T. A. Wadden. "Use of Dietary Supplements for Weight Loss in the United States: Results of a National Survey." *Obesity (Silver Spring)* 16, no. 4 (2008): 790–796.

Pratt, G. M., B. McLees, and W. J. Pories. "The ASBS Bariatric Surgery Centers of Excellence Program: A Blueprint for Quality Improvement." *Surgery for Obesity and Related Diseases* 2, no. 5 (2006): 497–503; discussion 503.

Purcell, K., P. Sumithran, L. A. Prendergast, C. J. Bouniu, E. Delbridge, and J. Proietto. "The Effect of Rate of Weight Loss on Long-Term Weight Management: A Randomised Controlled Trial." *The Lancet Diabetes & Endocrinology* 2, no. 12 (2014): 954–962.

Rubio, M. A., M. Gargallo, A. Isabel Millan, and B. Moreno. "Drugs in the Treatment of Obesity: Sibutramine, Orlistat and Rimonabant." *Public Health Nutrition* 10, no. 10A (2007): 1200–1205.

Rudd Center. "History of Menu Labeling Laws." 2011. Accessed August 1, 2011. http://yaleruddcenter.org/what_we_do.aspx?id=124.

Stagg-Elliott, V. "Is Obesity a Disease? Clinicians Disagree." 2006. Accessed January 6, 2009. http://www.ama-assn.org/amednews/2006/02/06/hlsa0206.htm.

Sumithran, P., and J. Proietto. "The Defence of Body Weight: A Physiological Basis for Weight Regain After Weight Loss." *Clinical Science* 124, no. 4 (2013): 231–241.

Thomas, J. G., D. S. Bond, S. Phelan, J. O. Hill, and R. R. Wing. "Weight-Loss Maintenance for 10 Years in the National Weight Control Registry." *The American Journal of Preventive Medicine* 46, no. 1 (2014): 17–23.

Tsai, A. G., and T. A. Wadden. "Systematic Review: An Evaluation of Major Commercial Weight Loss Programs in the United States." *Annals of Internal Medicine* 142, no. 1 (2005): 56–66.

United States Department of Agriculture (USDA). "Choose MyPlate.gov." 2014. Accessed December 18, 2014. http://www.choosemyplate.gov/.

United States Department of Agriculture (USDA). *U.S. Department of Agriculture Dietary Guidelines for Americans, 2015*. Washington, DC: U.S. Government Printing Office, 2015.

U.S. Department of Health and Human Services (USDHHS). "HHS Announces Revised Medicare Obesity Coverage Policy." 2004. Accessed May 12, 2011. http://www.hhs.gov/news/press/2004pres/20040715.html.

U.S. Department of Health and Human Services (USDHHS). *Physical Activity Guidelines for Americans*. Edited by U.S. Department of Health and Human

Services. Washington, DC: U.S. Department of Health and Human Services, 2009.

U.S. Department of Health and Human Services (USDHHS). "Healthy People 2020." 2011. U.S. Department of Health and Human Services. Accessed December 15, 2014. http://www.cdc.gov/nchs/healthy_people/hp2020.htm.

Wadden, T. A., and G. D. Foster. "Behavioral Treatment of Obesity." *Medical Clinics of North America* 84, no. 2 (2000): 441–461; vii.

Weintraub, M., J. D. Hasday, A. I. Mushlin, and D. H. Lockwood. "A Double-Blind Clinical Trial in Weight Control. Use of Fenfluramine and Phentermine Alone and in Combination." *Archives of Internal Medicine* 144, no. 6 (1984): 1143–1148.

Weintraub, M., P. R. Sundaresan, B. Schuster, G. Ginsberg, M. Madan, A. Balder, E. C. Stein, and L. Byrne. "Long-Term Weight Control Study." *Clinical Pharmacology and Therapeutics* 51, no. 5 (1992): 595–601.

West, J. A., and A. E. de Looy. "Weight Loss in Overweight Subjects Following Low-Sucrose or Sucrose-Containing Diets." *The International Journal of Obesity and Related Metabolic Disorders* 25, no. 8 (2001): 1122–1128.

The White House. "White House Task Force on Childhood Obesity Report to the President." 2010. Accessed July 20, 2011. http://www.letsmove.gov/white-house-task-force-childhood-obesity-report-president.

WIN. "Bariatric Surgery for Severe Obesity." 2011. National Institutes of Health. Accessed December 10, 2014. http://www.win.niddk.nih.gov/publications/gastric.htm#normaldigest.

Wing, R. R. "Behavioral Strategies to Improve Long-Term Weight Loss and Maintenance." *Medicine & Health Rhode Island* 82, no. 4 (1999): 123.

Woloshin, S., and L. M. Schwartz. "The New Weight-Loss Drugs, Lorcaserin and Phentermine-Topiramate: Slim Pickings?" *The Journal of the American Medical Association Internal Medicine* 174, no. 4 (2014): 615–619.

Wylie-Rosett, J. "Fat Substitutes and Health: An Advisory from the Nutrition Committee of the American Heart Association." *Circulation* 105, no. 23 (2002): 2800–2804.

Zheng, H., D. Tumin, and Z. Qian. "Obesity and Mortality Risk: New Findings from Body Mass Index Trajectories." *American Journal of Epidemiology* 178, no. 11 (2013):1591–1599.

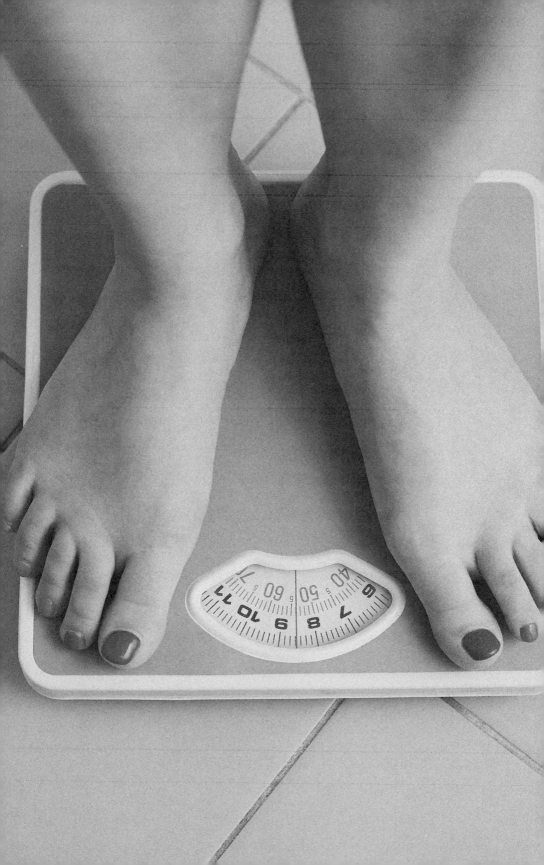

This chapter provides contributors with an opportunity to present their own personal views on a variety of issues related to obesity. Some essays describe individual experiences, while others provide updates on ongoing research.

Obesities

Nikhil V. Dhurandhar

It is no secret that two-thirds of the adults in the United States are either overweight or obese, and we are experiencing a global epidemic of obesity. It is also widely known that obesity is linked with numerous serious health conditions. The American Medical Association has recognized the seriousness of obesity and declared it a disease. The ongoing obesity research sponsored by various governmental and nongovernmental organizations and the campaigns to influence health-related policies and public health messages, all indicate that obesity is recognized as a key public health problem by various stakeholders. Why, then, are we unsuccessful in effectively preventing or treating obesity at the community or national level? There may be multiple reasons for our failure in effectively preventing or treating obesity. It is time to introspect and to learn from our experience, discontinue or modify the approaches that are

---

Obesity is more than just a number on the scale. It is a complex disease, and clinicians and researchers are still uncertain about effective prevention and treatment. Some answers may be found as we continue learning about individual success stories and testing new strategies. (Rostislav_sedlacek/Dreamstime.com)

unsuccessful, and to promote research and development of effective approaches.

Iterations of the message "eat less and move more" have been the mainstay of lifestyle modification-based obesity prevention and treatment approaches. Such studies have repeatedly demonstrated that a meaningful weight loss and maintenance is not achievable for the majority. This was best summarized by Dr. Albert Stunkard as follows: "Most persons will not stay in treatment for obesity. Of those who stay in treatment, most will not lose weight, and of those who do lose weight, most will regain it." The sad reality is that this quote, from nearly 60 years ago, is applicable even today. While good nutrition and exercise is good for the health of most individuals, a singular emphasis on these measures have not produced meaningful weight loss in adults or children. Traditionally, the bar for measuring success of a weight loss program has been set very low. A weight loss of 5 percent of body weight is considered adequate to improve health. Despite the low bar, in most behavioral weight loss programs, a majority of the participants do not lose even 5 percent weight. Moreover, recent studies have questioned the adequacy of 5 percent weight loss for improving health. Some surgeries for obesity yield much greater weight loss, which has allowed a closer examination of the relationship of weight loss and the improvement in comorbidities. It appears that weight losses much larger than 5 percent may be needed to obtain substantial health benefits of weight loss. Thus, creating a negative energy balance by reducing energy intake and increasing energy expenditure may be sound in theory for obesity management. However, in reality, this approach has not provided promising results. A candid and critical evaluation is needed to determine the underlying reasons and to explore any alternatives.

The typical weight loss recommendations to 'eat less and move more' seem to have some major drawbacks. First, they seem to presume this behavior to be completely under volitional control, and hence willfully modifiable. This may not be the case, based on the role of physiology, environment, and genetics in energy intake and expenditure. For instance, the response of PYY3–36, a hormone secreted by the gut in response to food intake, is delayed in individuals suffering from obesity. This delayed onset of satiety may expose the person to greater energy intake. Studies have uncovered many such examples of non-volitional regulation of energy stores. Even if the influence of non-volitional factors is discounted, volitional regulation alone of energy intake or expenditure is not adequate to induce a meaningful and sustained weight loss in individuals predisposed to obesity. As we know, one big meal does not cause obesity and one small meal does not cure obesity. A sustained and chronic negative energy balance is needed for a sustained weight loss. This demand for sustained long-term change imposes a highly unrealistic expectation. For example, similar to eating, breathing rate is also under some volitional control. Hence, in theory, it is possible to voluntarily reduce the rate of breathing for a while. It is, however, near impossible to voluntarily continue a subnormal rate of breathing for months or years on end. Similarly, the need to control energy intake or expenditure long term makes it unsustainable for approaches that exclusively depend on behavioral changes.

There is an increased awareness for the need to supplement lifestyle modification to increase compliance with weight loss diets. The U.S. Food and Drug Administration (FDA) has recently approved five drugs to combat obesity, which are expected to empower a person to adhere to a weight loss regimen. They are a supplement and not a substitute to lifestyle modification for reducing obesity. Like any drug, these drugs have the potential for adverse effects. They are effective only when consumed; weight gain can result if the drugs are discontinued. Also, the efficacy of obesity drugs varies considerably among individuals. Hence, the availability of a larger number of obesity drugs would create more options for physicians to select an effective treatment most suited for an individual. Unfortunately, very few drug options exist today for treating obesity. This is illustrated well by hypertension medications. Several dozen antihypertensive medications allow a physician to select the optimal medication for an individual. Similarly, a larger number of obesity medications with varying mechanism of action are needed to manage obesity. This is also applicable to some surgical approaches advanced for obesity management. Many types of bariatric surgery procedures are superior to other weight loss approaches in terms of weight lost and maintenance, particularly for those with a high degree of obesity, which has otherwise remained mostly intractable. Importantly, harnessing the underlying mechanism of bariatric surgical procedures is needed to develop approaches that can reproduce the benefits nonsurgically.

Currently, obesity treatment is mainly limited to lifestyle modification, obesity drugs, and surgery. In general, the potential for wide-scale applicability of these approaches decreases from lifestyle modification to obesity surgery, whereas the efficacy increases in the reverse order. Prevention and treatment approaches that are both effective as well as widely applicable are needed. The current approaches primarily aim at inducing a negative energy balance by modifying energy intake and/or activity. Perhaps, it is important to consider the upstream factors that lead to a positive energy balance in the first place. Many studies have recognized additional putative contributors to the obesity epidemic, including sleep debt, certain infections, gut microbiota, maternal-fetal environment, changes in ambient temperatures, assortative mating, endocrine disrupters, and other environmental influences. It may be highly important to consider this multifactorial etiology of obesity for developing cause-specific prevention and treatment strategies for obesity—an approach that has received little attention.

Similar to the term "cancer," the term "obesity" is inadequate to convey the contribution of multiple causative factors. The etiology of cancer includes smoking, radiation, viruses, genetics, and several other factors. Each type of cancer may need a cause-specific prevention and treatment approach. Similarly, instead of "obesity," the term "obesities" may better describe the multifactorial etiology and may guide the development of cause-specific prevention and treatment. For example, sleep hygiene will have to be addressed, if sleep debt is contributing to an individual's obesity. If viral infections, such as certain human adenoviruses, have the potential to influence body weight, a virus-specific vaccine may be needed to prevent that subtype of obesity. Of the putative contributors of obesity, some may not be modifiable. Nonetheless, a comprehensive understanding of the causes of obesity is needed for developing cause-specific prevention and treatment approaches. Such an approach may be more effective than the currently employed "blanket treatment" of obesity, which seldom considers the above mentioned putative contributors of obesity.

In summary, although inadequate, lifestyle modification, obesity drugs, and surgery are the best available treatments for obesity at present. While we continue to offer them to those suffering from obesity, it is important to acknowledge their limitations, and to recognize the need to develop more effective and widely applicable approaches. The research breakthrough may not come from repeating or incrementally modifying the approaches repeatedly shown to be marginally effective. Cause-specific prevention and treatment is a concept commonly used for addressing cancer or jaundice or many other diseases, but it is underexplored in the field of obesity. Developing such approaches will require a thorough understanding of the putative as well as hitherto unknown causes of obesity. Using the term "obesities" instead of "obesity" may best convey this message.

References

Dhurandhar, N. V. "A Framework for Identification of Infections That Contribute to Human Obesity." *The Lancet Infectious Diseases* 11, no. 12 (2011): 963–969.

Dhurandhar, N. V. "When Commonsense Does Not Make Sense." *International Journal of Obesity* 36, no. 10 (2012): 1332–1333.

McAllister, E. J., N. V. Dhurandhar, S. W. Keith, L. J. Aronne, J. Barger, M. Baskin, R. M. Benca, et al. "Ten Putative Contributors to the Obesity Epidemic." *Critical Reviews in Food Science and Nutrition* 49, no. 10 (2009): 868–913.

Shaya, F. T., D. Flores, C. M. Gbarayor, and J. Wang. "School-Based Obesity Interventions: A Literature Review." *Journal of School Health* 78, no. 4 (2008): 189–196.

Sjostrom, C. D., T. Lystig, and A. K. Lindroos. "Impact of Weight Change, Secular Trends and Ageing on Cardiovascular Risk Factors: 10-Year Experiences from the Sos Study." *International Journal of Obesity* 35, no. 11 (2011): 1413–1420.

Stunkard A. J. "The Management of Obesity." *New York State Journal of Medicine* 58 (1958): 79–87.

Wadden, T. A. "Treatment of Obesity by Moderate and Severe Caloric Restriction. Results of Clinical Research Trials." *Annals of Internal Medicine* 119, no. 7 Pt 2 (1993): 688–693.

Zinn, A. R. "Unconventional Wisdom about the Obesity Epidemic." *The American Journal of Medical Sciences* 340, no. 6 (2010): 481–491.

Dr. Nikhil V. Dhurandhar is professor and chair of the department of Nutritional Sciences at Texas Tech University, Lubbock, Texas, USA. He was president of The Obesity Society for 2014–2015 and an editor of the International Journal of Obesity. *As a physician and nutritional biochemist, he has been involved with obesity treatment and research for over 20 years and has treated over 10,000 patients for obesity using lifestyle therapy as well as pharmacological approaches. Dr. Dhurandhar and colleagues were the first to identify adenoviruses that cause obesity in animals and show an association with obesity in humans. Dr. Dhurandhar believes that simple explanations for causes of obesity are inadequate and novel approaches are required for its effective management.*

No More Obesity

Rajiv Narayan

Until age 18, I had been obese my entire life. I could see in old family pictures that I had been thinner once, but that time had passed so long ago that for most of my life I had only known what it was like to be fat. But that changed quickly. Within the first two years of college, I managed to lose about 100 pounds.

While I was losing the weight, I grew to be very interested in obesity as an issue—I obsessed over what role I played in this "obesity epidemic" I was reading all about, and how it was that I managed to lose weight when all the research I read suggested that the odds were against me. Some part of me wanted to find the answer to these questions because I thought my weight loss was too good to be true, too good to last more than a couple months before I would inevitably gain it all back. Another part of me, a part that would grow over time, realized that my weight loss success was not so much a success as it was a massive privilege. I had the privilege of finding the right intervention for my own type of obesity. It used to be that I would tell others I lost weight by way of disciplined diet and exercise. That is not untrue, but it is at best incomplete and simplistic.

Now, when others ask how I managed to lose so much weight, my answer is longer. First, I had the privilege of moving 100 miles away to attend college. This space provided me with a fresh start, a chance to make new habits, break old ones, and slough off what others had expected of me. Second, I went to a campus that required constant physical activity. My dorm was right across the street from the campus gym. My college was recognized for having the country's most bike-friendly campus. Third, I had a tremendous amount of social and economic support. I was not struggling to make ends meet or balancing too many responsibilities. All I was expected to focus on was school, and I had all the free time leftover to focus on my body. And, so it stands as all too clear that the factors that contributed to my weight loss could not be recommended for most others.

All of this is to say that I learned there was not one obesity, to which I was a part of, but many obesities, each with their own causes, symptoms, challenges, and inflection points. If we are to solve the obesity epidemic in the coming decades, that moment will come when we recognize that there is no obesity epidemic. There is instead an epidemic of many obesities, the solution for which will depend on matching lived experience, research, and intervention to the many forms this health condition takes.

To conceive of many obesities is not a new idea, and certainly not one unique to obesity itself (Kopelman 2007). Models and methods of productive disease subtyping can be found in the many types of diabetes and asthma, to say nothing of cancer (Field 2013). Having the ability to distinguish between allergic, nonallergic, occupational, and exercise-induced asthma or pre-diabetes, gestational diabetes, type 1 diabetes and type 2 diabetes has allowed researchers and clinicians to develop interventions that fit more closely the ailment they are treating, thus improving outcomes for patients. To go further, misdiagnosing the type of diabetes can be disastrous to a patient.

So, how will obesity become a series of obesities? So far, researchers have been hard at work identifying meaningful differences in physiological mechanisms, socioeconomic status, racial and ethnic background, life history, and treatment efficacy. The results are sprawling.

Someone with centripetal obesity needs perhaps a more urgent treatment plan than an obese person with a more even distribution of body fat (Després 2006). The group of obesities termed "infectobesity" for their link to viruses, bacteria, and other pathogens may be best treated with targeted medicines (Pasarica 2007). Being able to scale BMI to account for different risk ratios in different ethnic groups is crucial to addressing comorbidities with the appropriate vigilance (Misra 2009). Moreover, even where physiology is not clinically distinguishable, there are meaningful differences for treatment with respect to socioeconomic status and life history. Even at the same BMI, the obese, low-income single parent with three children and two jobs has a very different embodied experience of obesity than her peer of middle-income status in a two-parent household (Warin 2008). The need for a caloric deficit may be imperative in each of these cases, but the pathway to getting there will vary by type of obesity.

For obesity to be subtyped effectively, it will be important to not only study the different causal mechanisms of obesity, but also what differences exist within those groups who do manage to lose a significant amount of weight. A landmark study to this effect has already begun in the analysis of the National Weight Control Registry (NWCR). The NWCR is an observational study of more than 5,000 participants who have each demonstrated long-term weight loss maintenance of at least 30 pounds for at least one year. As the registry approaches a life of two decades, researchers have begun to identify some commonalities in sustainable weight loss maintenance, such constant weight and diet monitoring, low-carbohydrate diets, and never missing breakfast. Ogden went further to demonstrate a cluster analysis of NWCR participants, showing groupings of shared weight loss biographies (Ogden 2012).

The first cluster of participants, accounting for just over half of the registry, were identified as exercise conscious and satisfied with their weight. The second cluster accounted for over a quarter of participants, and came to rely on many resources in their continuous struggle to maintain weight loss. They are more likely to have greater stress, more likely to be depressed. The third cluster, representing just over 12 percent of participants, lost a great deal of weight on their first try, were typically obese as children, and experienced the fewest challenges in weight loss maintenance. The last cluster of the final 10 percent of participants is older in age. They are less likely to undertake exercise, but compensate for this by eating less. They tend to exhibit more health problems, too.

Knowing the etiologies of different obesities is not enough; studies like this one show that it is valuable for treatment follow-up and personal long-term weight loss maintenance to develop a sense of the kind of journey a person's weight loss is likely to take.

Just as a fracturing of many obesities creates opportunities for creative and strategic engagement, it will also amplify several practical and political challenges. Because the causes and experience of obesity are deeply entrenched in the life course of a person, integrative healthcare teams are needed to deliver comprehensive care. Having the ability to typify obesities will require clinicians to develop a plan with the patient that could incorporate many actors, from a dietician to social workers, community health workers to family members, diabetes educators, and more. Though the need for complicated care will impose a burden on resources and a challenge for effective cross-communication, it is crucial.

Also pressing is the political reality of many obesities. The obesity epidemic currently attracts a mass of resources and attention, from philanthropic investment to research grants to government action and media hype. That all obesities have been able to fly under the banner of a unitary epidemic has been useful for advocates. But when obesities begin to diverge, some patient populations will have more clout than others, and so it is possible these groups will command more resources and consequently better treatments for their type. Already, epidemiological studies are showing that obesity policies have yielded better outcomes for higher income communities as well as predominantly white populations, while low-income communities and communities of color continue to see high or higher obesity rates (Levi 2014). Should the subtyping of obesities round up underprivileged patient populations, it will be all the more important to work with these groups and advocate for just as much prudent research attention and treatment access, not to mention the need for systemic changes that address the many structural oppressions that can promote obesity. There currently is and will continue to be a need for equity in obesity policy.

Most important of all, a future of many obesities will place upon us the need to recognize and respect the diversity of patients. Realizing that my obesity was plain different from others was not isolating. Even with multiple obesities, we can stand in solidarity for thoughtful care.

References

Despres, J. P., and I. Lemieux. "Abdominal Obesity and Metabolic Syndrome." *Nature* 444, no. 7121 (2006): 881–887.

Field, A. E., C. A. Camargo, Jr., and S. Ogino.. "The Merits of Subtyping Obesity: One Size Does Not Fit All." *Journal of the American Medical Association* 310, no. 20 (2013): 2147–2148.

Kopelman, P., S. A. Jebb, and B. Butland. "Executive Summary: Foresight 'Tackling Obesities: Future Choices' Project." *Obesity Reviews* 8, Suppl. 1 (2007): vi–ix.

Levi, J., Segal, L. M. and Gadola, E. *The State of Obesity: Better Policies for a Healthier America 2014*. Edited by the Trust for America's Health. Washington, DC, 2014.

Misra, A., P. Chowbey, B. M. Makkar, N. K. Vikram, J. S. Wasir, D. Chadha, S. R. Joshi, S. Sadikot, R. Gupta, S. Gulati, Y. P. Munjal, and Group Concensus. "Consensus Statement for Diagnosis of Obesity, Abdominal Obesity and the Metabolic Syndrome for Asian Indians and Recommendations for Physical Activity, Medical and Surgical Management." *The Journal of the Association of Physicians of India* 57 (Feb. 2009): 163–170.

Rajiv Narayan entered the obesity field after losing 100 lbs. He completed his M.Sc. in Medical Anthropology at the University of Oxford as a Rotary Ambassadorial Scholar and is currently at the Center for Health Equity at the New York City Department of Health and Mental Hygiene.

Obesity Prevention: The Bathroom Scale Model—A Perspective on Weight Reduction, Weight Regain Prevention, and Obesity Prevention

Barbara Hansen

Most weight reduction studies involving pharmaceutical or behavioral interventions in patients with overweight or obesity have had small to modest success in producing weight losses of 10–20 pounds, sometimes cited as 4–6 percent weight loss. These studies invariably recommend reduced calorie intake and increased physical activity. Patients are generally positive about their reduced weight. Nevertheless, weight regain remains the near universal finding.

While some attribute this to return of bad habits, thus blaming the patient for his own recidivism, as a physiologist and researcher of appetite regulation in nonhuman primates, my view of this phenomenon is that it is physiological regulation of appetite and body weight that ultimately and nearly always wins out. Just as the human body regulates its temperature within narrow limits despite wide ranges of ambient temperature, the human body (and in fact, the nonhuman primate body and most other mammals) also regulates body weight within a narrow range. That range, based purely on observations of both humans and monkeys, has a strong tendency to increase in "middle age" as it gradually and slowly increases in humans from age 30 to 60 years and in monkeys from age 10 to 20 years. Later in life, there is a tendency to show some decline in weight unrelated to overt diseases. This occurs in humans over the period 60–90 years and in monkeys over the period 20–30 years. This naturally occurring lifelong weight gain and loss trajectory has proven to be very robust and difficult to alter significantly.

Why is this and what can be done to alter this course? It is easy to attribute these observations to genetics, and therefore unalterable (at least for now). But on the other hand, a small number of persons do seem to be successful, including those currently being followed on the National Weight Control Registry (individuals who have lost at least 30 pounds and maintained a weight loss of at least 30 pounds for one year or more). Those on the Registry have most frequently attributed their success to a regimen high in exercise, although the validity of this attribution has been questioned. The dose effect of exercise as a weight loss agent or as a weight regain prevention agent seems to be very limiting for most patients. Thus, if a patient is consistently adherent to an increased physical activity level of 30 minutes or more of moderate exercise on 5 or more days per week, as might be prescribed by a physician, the net effect might result in an increased expenditure of about 600 calories per week. In that same week, the caloric intake of this sample patient might amount to more than 9,000 calories, and furthermore, increased exercise might be met with increased food intake in an apparent compensatory action of the body regulatory system within the normal range of activity (Mayer 1954).

We are forced, therefore, to reconsider the issue of long-term sustainable calorie restriction. In this regard, the nonhuman primates provide some views that might enlighten. Concerning the successful reduction of body weight by substantial calorie reduction (reduced food availability), obese monkeys have lost greater than 20 percent of their body weight during weight reduction experiments. They also have had the ability to retain that lower body weight level for up to 2 years, providing that, however, a new level of calorie restraint is imposed. Stable body weight at a weight reduced level is achieved at a calorie intake level of about 30–40 percent lower than the prior steady state intake level during ad libitum feeding, of course depending on the amount of weight lost. The point is that after weight reduction it is necessary to consume a lower calorie intake to maintain a stable weight. There is some evidence that, after body weight is reduced, metabolism is more efficient; that is, a body uses fewer calories per kilogram lean body mass than was used in the preweight reduction phase (DeLany 1999). Rudy Leibel and colleagues noted this in patients who had lost weight intentionally (Leibel 1995), and we have confirmed this in nonhuman primates in whom every calorie ingested was measured. We have produced more than 20 percent weight loss in obese monkeys and have stabilized them for either 2 months or 2 years at their reduced level of body weight, simply by adjusting the calories available to each individual monkey on a weekly basis to maintain stable reduced weight. At the end of either 2 months or 2 years of stable reduced weight, the animals were returned to ad libitum food availability. Perhaps predictably, the physiology took over. The bad "habits" were not permanently overcome (although there is no evidence that bad habits ever caused obesity in either humans or monkeys); weight regain inevitably occurred in all monkeys and they returned at least to or beyond their starting weights. It should be added that the composition of the diet was considered optimally healthy: high in fiber, low in total fat, and low in saturated fat content. The palatability and composition of the diet was kept constant throughout these long-term studies. Similar regain of induced weight loss has been regularly reported in humans, as well. Interestingly, this gain was achieved with minimal or no "overeating"; that is, no ingestion of greater calories per kilogram lean body mass or total calories per day than had been taken voluntarily in the run-in baseline ad libitum feeding period. It seems that we must accept that the body "knows" when it is at a lower than "running" level and gradually fixes that problem if there is food availability.

In a politically correct manner, we have, therefore, sought behavioral changes to slow or prevent the middle-aged gain in weight (or in pediatric groups, to slow the rate of weight gain) under the belief system that it might be easier to keep weight off than to take it off once it has been gained. How does that work in monkeys? We have carried out a study of more than 20 years in adult rhesus monkeys who were "weight clamped" at an age of about 10 years, equivalent to about 30 years in humans. In monkeys, maintained in a laboratory setting, this was relatively easy to achieve by weighing each individual monkey once per week, and accordingly adjusting the daily calorie allotment for each monkey depending on whether weight had been gained or lost over the past week. In this way, monkeys were maintained well past middle age at the weight they had been when they were in early adulthood. Because the weight was required to remain stable by this weekly adjustment, we refer to this as a weight clamp. This approach recognized that one size does not fit all, and that despite being similar in body weight, the calorie requirements of each monkey differed. Had we clamped calories provided to be the same and steady for all monkeys, instead of choosing to clamp weight, some of the monkeys would have lost weight and others gained weight on the same number of calories per day.

Now, for the bad news: despite years of maintenance at a steady weight and prevention of increase in adipose tissue, when tested in acute short refeeding tests, the monkeys were and remained hungry! They ate faster and more calories per minute in their calorie restrained condition, and had not adapted to it. Appetite regulation remained unimpaired and hefty. From these studies, we conclude that long-term calorie restraint does not "fix" the system and does not result in lower steady state eating behavior or reduced physiological appetite regulation. Long-term restrained calorie intake, at whatever level is needed to sustain the lost weight level, is necessary to achieve long-term prevention of either regain of lost weight or initial natural gain in weight.

For humans, even those with excellent nutritional knowledge and experience, the challenge of calculating the calories in a mixed meal on a dinner plate and, more importantly, calculating all the calories ingested in a day is beyond the ability of any of us, except under defined formula intakes. If, as I believe, we cannot successfully calculate and measure our own food intake in calories per day consumed, what then can we monitor? There seems to be only one answer to this question:

the daily recording of the bathroom scale weight. It tells the truth about whether reduced calorie intake has actually been continually achieved. Daily weighing allows one to see the inherent variability in the measurement from day to day and to adjust intakes to prevent weigh regain (or to achieve weight loss initially). Unfortunately, despite multiple claims, there is no one way to restrain calories either for weight reduction or weight loss maintenance; thus, whatever works is the best approach. Any approach that moves the scale downward gradually in the overweight, or holds steady the reduced weight, is acceptable (within reason, of course). Most important is the acceptance that the scale does not lie, and the intake is indeed too much if during attempts at weight loss it is not occurring, or if recidivism post weight loss is occurring.

Viva la bathroom scale! Out with the kitchen scale!

References

DeLany, J. P., B.C. Hansen, N. L. Bodkin, J. Hannah, and G. A. Bray. "Long-Term Calorie Restriction Reduces Energy Expenditure in Aging Monkeys." *The Journals of Gerontology Series A: Biological Sciences and Medical Sciences* 54, no. 1 (1999): B5–B11; discussion B12–B3.

Leibel, R. L., M. Rosenbaum, and J. Hirsch. "Changes in Energy Expenditure Resulting from Altered Body Weight." *New England Journal of Medicine* 332, no. 10 (1995): 621–628.

Mayer, J., N. B. Marshall, J. J. Vitale, J. H. Christensen, M. B. Mashayekhi, and F. J. Stare. "Exercise, Food Intake and Body Weight in Normal Rats and Genetically Obese Adult Mice." *American Journal of Physiology* 177, no. 3 (1954): 544–548.

Dr. Barbara Hansen is the director of the Obesity, Diabetes, and Aging Research Center of the College of Medicine and Professor of

Internal Medicine and Pediatrics at the University of South Florida, Tampa. Her research has addressed the physiological, cellular, and molecular defects underlying the development and prevention of obesity and diabetes in humans and nonhuman primate models. Dr. Hansen is a member of the Institute of Medicine of the National Academy of Sciences. She has served as president of the North American Association for the Study of Obesity (The Obesity Society) and as the first president of the International Association for the Study of Obesity (IASO).

Pros and Cons of Dietary Supplements for Weight Management

Kelly Morrow

Dietary supplements for weight management are among the most popular supplements on the market. According to consumer reports, one in four Americans use these supplements, and the industry grew 11.6 percent in 2013. In my experience as a clinical dietitian and as a dietary supplement sales representative, I have encountered many people who use supplements for weight management. Some want and edge in the process. Others THINK they will not have to exercise as much or to restrict food. Some want to jump-start their metabolism or suppress their appetite. Anything to make the weight loss easier and less painful!

There are a few dietary supplements that have some scientific evidence showing they can be helpful, but for most, the evidence for any efficacy is lacking. Many weight loss supplements have only been studied in animals or in small populations. A large percentage of supplements marketed for weight loss do nothing. Probably, one of the best studied supplements is caffeine, either as a chemical or as a part of some herb. Although it can increase weight loss and suppress the appetite, it does so at a health-related price. In many people, caffeine can raise blood pressure and cause insomnia and anxiety.

Dietary Supplement Labeling

By definition, dietary supplements are meant to "add nutritional value to the diet," although many people take dietary supplements to prevent disease, promote weight loss, build muscle, and other medical reasons. Dietary supplement labels are allowed to contain "structure function claims" that are intended to describe how the supplement could affect the structure or function of the body such as "maintains healthy metabolism" or "support for appetite regulation." To further illustrate the difference between a drug claim and a structure function claim, the label must also include the statement "This claim has not been reviewed by the FDA. This product is not intended to diagnose, treat, cure, or prevent any disease." Many critics feel that structure function claims are misleading and too similar to a drug claim. The Federal Trade Commission (FTC) is responsible for investigating false and misleading label claims and sends warning letters to companies that push the boundaries. Weight loss supplements that make claims about quick weight loss, herbal alternatives to prescription drugs, and other quick fixes or "secret scientific breakthroughs" should obviously be looked at with extreme caution. Consumers, healthcare providers, and industry watchdogs can report misleading label claims to the FTC.

What Are the Risks of Taking Supplements for Weight Management?

Aside from dubious marketing claims aimed at a vulnerable population, weight loss supplements are often contaminated with illegal substances, including pharmaceutical drugs and other banned and unregulated ingredients (FDA 2014; Cohen 2014). According to the FDA, the three most risky dietary supplement categories include those used for sexual enhancement, body building (ergogenic), and weight loss. A recent analysis of dietary supplement recalls showed that these three categories alone made up 98 percent of dietary supplement recalls due to class 1 drug adulteration (Harel 2013). Perhaps, more alarming is the report that up to 67 percent of the contaminated weight loss supplements, 85 percent of body building, and 20 percent of sexual enhancement supplements are still available and sold after being recalled (Cohen 2014).

The main reason this problem persists has to do with the way dietary supplements are regulated by the FDA. Unlike pharmaceutical drugs, dietary supplements are regulated as a subcategory of food and are not approved before they are put on the market. According to the law that regulates dietary supplements, the Dietary Supplement Health and Education Act (DSHEA), supplement companies are responsible for following the FDA manufacturing and safety guidelines, but are not required to submit proof of compliance before selling their products. The FDA bears the burden of proving a supplement is unsafe and does this by performing spot checks on manufacturing facilities, responding to tips from consumers, healthcare providers, retailers, and from adverse event reports (Harel 2013). In the system that exists now, the FDA does not have the resources to adequately remove recalled products from the market, especially with the complexity of supplement distribution, including internet sales and small retail operations.

Even if a dietary supplement does not contain illegal ingredients, other quality issues remain. Many supplement manufacturers do not adequately test raw materials or finished products to ensure they are meeting label claim. The FDA reports that up to 70 percent of audited supplement manufacturers are not in full compliance with FDA-mandated Good Manufacturing Procedures. The most common violations include failure to adequately test raw materials and finished products, failure to keep adequate records, and contamination of products with unintended or banned ingredients. Several products have been banned or have had warnings issued by the FDA. *Ephedra sinica* and DMAA both have been promoted as weight loss supplements, but have been banned due to numerous cardiovascular complications and deaths. In 2013, a fat-burning supplement called OxyElite Pro caused cases of liver failure and hepatitis due to adulteration of its formula.

Despite these problems, there are relatively few serious adverse events (hospitalization, disability, or death) that can be clearly linked to dietary supplements. This may be due to a lack of adequate reporting of adverse events and also due to the fact that many people with adverse events have complex medical histories and are taking multiple medications and supplements simultaneously. Anyone who experiences adverse events related to dietary supplements can file a report with the FDA MedWatch program.

How to Choose a Quality Supplement

Consumers of dietary supplements must be vigilant in order to ensure they are taking safe and high-quality products, especially when taking products designed for weight loss. Several companies exist to help consumers choose quality products. Consumer Lab (www.consumerlabs.com) is one of the best known resources. Scientists pull dietary supplements off store shelves randomly, analyze them in certified labs, and publish the report. For a small annual fee, subscribers can find out if their supplement brand meets label claim or is contaminated in any way.

The U.S. Pharmacopeia, Natural Products Association, and the National Sanitation Foundation all offer third-party testing on dietary supplements to ensure they are in compliance with the FDA. If a dietary supplement company has paid for this service, the product has a stamp on the label denoting the organization that has done third-party testing.

Many of the major label brand dietary supplements sold in health food stores and mass market retailers are of high quality and are safe. The biggest problems usually come from obscure brands, especially if bought off the internet and products sold in the riskiest supplement categories—weight loss, ergogenic/body building, and sexual enhancement.

Where to Learn More about Supplements

The Office of Dietary Supplements (http://ods.od.nih.gov) was commissioned as part of the DSHEA as a resource for consumers and health care providers to find credible information about dietary supplements. This free site contains technical data sheets, FAQ's, and FDA warnings and recalls.

The Natural Medicines Comprehensive Database (www. naturaldatabase.therapeuticresearch.com) is the most comprehensive resource for healthcare providers to access current information about use, dosage, forms, drug nutrient interactions, and contraindications associated with dietary supplements. For an annual fee, subscribers can get access from any computer, tablet, or mobile device.

References

Cohen, P.A., G. Maller, R. DeSouza, and J. Neal-Kababick. "Presence of Banned Drugs in Dietary Supplements Following FDA Recalls." *Journal of the American Medical Association* 312, no. 16 (2014): 1691–1693.

FDA. "Beware of Products Promising Miracle Weight Loss." 2015. Food and Drug Administration. Accessed January 6, 2015. http://www.fda.gov/ForConsumers/ ConsumerUpdates/ucm246742.htm.

Harel, Z., S. Harel, R. Wald, M. Mamdani, and C.M. Bell. "The Frequency and Characteristics of Dietary Supplement Recalls in the United States." *Journal of the American Medical Association Intern Med* 173 no.10 (2013): 926–928.

Kelly Morrow, MS, RDN, is a registered dietitian nutritionist, associate professor in the Department of Nutrition and Exercise Science at Bastyr University, and nutrition clinic coordinator at the Bastyr Center for Natural Health.

Low-Calorie Sweeteners and Weight Management

Lyn O'Brien Nabors

Low-calorie sweeteners (LCS) have long been of interest to scientists, regulators, and consumers alike. As a group, LCS is one of, if not, the most studied group of food ingredients. Consumers like sweets, and there is historical evidence that humans have always had a preference for sweets and research shows that the desire for sweets is inborn. People understand the purpose of sweeteners, as opposed to their knowledge or interest in emulsifiers and antioxidants, for example. There are currently several low/no calorie sweeteners available for use in the United States, including acesulfame K, advantame, aspartame, monk fruit, neotame, saccharin, stevia, and sucralose. Cyclamate is approved in over 100 countries, although not currently in the United States.

Some have claimed that LCS perpetuate a desire for sweet foods and beverages and stimulate appetite—leading to increased intake and weight gain. Such speculation is not supported by science. Conversely, scientific research shows that LCS do not stimulate appetite or food intake and do not result in weight gain. LCS and reduced-calorie products containing LCS may result in reduced caloric intake and weight. They are not drugs that make one lose weight but tools to assist in weight management, in conjunction with reduced caloric intake and increased activity.

Especially with the "obesity epidemic," the usefulness of LCS in efforts to lose or maintain weight has been questioned. The idea that their use could result in weight gain is illogical since they add no calories to the diet. It is duly noted that, if one chooses to drink a diet soda in order to eat pecan pie, weight loss is unlikely to occur. Although all LCS provide essentially no calories, they differ in other ways such as chemical composition and sweetening power. Therefore, efforts to lump them together and imply that as a group they result in weight gain has no basis in science.

For example, aspartame is most frequently used as the "poster child" by proponents of the "low-calorie sweeteners make you gain weight theory" (as well as other equally unscientific claims). Aspartame is made up of two amino acids (aspartic acid and phenylalanine) and methanol. When digested, aspartame breaks down into small amounts of these components, which are used in the same way by the body as when they are derived from common foods. A serving of nonfat milk provides about 6 times more phenylalanine and 13 times more aspartic acid compared to an equivalent amount of diet soda sweetened with aspartame alone. A serving of tomato juice provides six times more methanol compared to an equal amount of diet soda sweetened with aspartame. Neither aspartame nor its components accumulate in the body.

Numerous studies have been conducted over the past 30-plus years to examine LCS in relation to body weight. There is now a significant human database, so it is difficult to understand why some continue to conduct and promote animal studies on the issue. A meta-analysis of 15 randomized controlled human trials (RCTs) and 9 prospective cohort studies on LCS and body weight and composition was published in 2014. The researchers concluded that "data from RCTs, which provide the highest quality of evidence for the potentially causal effects of LCS intake, indicated that substituting LCS options for their regular-calorie versions results in modest weight loss, and may be a useful dietary tool to improve compliance with weight loss or weight maintenance plans" (Miller and Perez 2014).

Furthermore, in 2014, results of an online survey administered to members of the National Weight Control Registry, which is made up of individuals who have lost 13.6 kg or more and maintained the loss for more than a year, were published. The objective of the study was to evaluate prevalence of and strategies of low/no calorie beverage (LNCSB) consumption in successful weight loss maintainers. Researchers concluded that regular consumption of LNCSB is common in successful weight loss maintainers. Among reasons given for their use is to limit total energy intake (Catenacci et al. 2014).

Interestingly, research shows that those using LCS have a better quality diet. In a recently published study, diet quality was examined using the U.S. Department of Agriculture's Healthy Eating Index (HEI 2005), a measure of diet quality that assesses conformance to federal dietary guidance. National Health and Nutrition Examination Surveys (NHANES) from 1999 to 2000, 2001–2002, 2003–2004, 2005–2006, and 2007–2008, which provide data on dietary intakes and multiple health indicators, were analyzed. LCS use was associated with higher HEI 2005 scores (higher HEI subscores for vegetables, whole grains, and low-fat dairy), lower consumption of empty calories, less smoking, and more physical activity (Drewnowski and Rehm 2014).

Health professionals agree that LCS may assist with weight management. For example, a 2011 statement of the American Heart Association and American Diabetes Association concludes that when used judiciously, LCS may help with weight loss or control, and could also have beneficial metabolic effects. However, the statement also points out that potential benefits will not be completely realized if there is a compensatory increase in energy intake from other sources (Gardner et al. 2012).

The vast majority of the research on the safety and use of LCS is sponsored by industry. The petitioner for the use of a new sweetener is required to provide studies in support of the sweetener's safety. Who, other than a company expecting to benefit from approval, would be interested in or willing to spend the millions of dollars on studies necessary for approval? It follows that studies on the benefits of the LCS would also be sponsored by industry. Unfortunately, the validity of industry-funded research has been brought into question and greater scrutiny of industry sponsored has been suggested. As a result, academicians evaluated the association of the funding source and quality or reporting of long-term obesity randomized clinical trials. Sixty-seven percent of the 63 randomized clinical trials were industry funded. Industry sponsoring was associated with a higher quality of reporting score in long-term weight loss studies compared to nonindustry-funded trials (Thomas et al. 2008).

Also pertinent to the review of scientific literature is the issue of researcher bias, which can result in a misleading representation of data. Cope and Allison (2010) demonstrated that a "white hat" bias may exist in obesity research. This bias refers to the tendency to distort research findings, if it is perceived to serve righteous ends. These scientists examined ways in which researchers writing reports on new studies referenced two previous studies, which reported effects of sugar-sweetened beverages on body weight. An analysis of 206 papers citing the two studies found that the study results were described in a misleading manner (e.g., exaggerating the strength of the evidence that reducing sugar-sweetened drink consumption reduced weight or obesity) more than 66 percent of the time. Cope and Allison also reported that data showing statistically significant nutritive-sweetened beverage outcomes was more likely to be published, and when data did not show sugar-sweetened drinks to have the desired outcome, it was less likely to be published. They also noted that this publishing bias appears to be only for nonindustry-funded research and all industry-funded studies seem "to exceed a minimal level of precision."

LCS can play an important role in reducing caloric intake. Foods and beverages containing LCS, reduced in sugar and/ or calories, provide good tasting options, significantly lower in calories than their full calorie counterparts. Numerous studies support the benefits of these products and the supporting studies should be judged on the merits of the study, not on the funding source.

References

Catenacci, V. A., Z. Pan, J. G. Thomas, L. G. Ogden, S. A. Roberts, H. R. Wyatt, R. R. Wing, and J. O. Hill. "Low/No Calorie Sweetened Beverage Consumption in the National

Weight Control Registry." *Obesity (Silver Spring)* 22 no. 10 (2014): 2244–2251.

Cope, M. B., and D. B. Allison. "White Hat Bias: Examples of Its Presence in Obesity Research and a Call for Renewed Commitment to Faithfulness in Research Reporting." *International Journal of Obesity* 34, no. 1 (2010): 84–88; discussion 83.

Drewnowski, A., and C. D. Rehm. "Consumption of Low-Calorie Sweeteners among U.S. Adults is Associated with Higher Healthy Eating Index (HEI 2005) Scores and More Physical Activity." *Nutrients* 6, no. 10 (2014): 4389–4403.

Gardner, C., J. Wylie-Rosett, S. S. Gidding, L. M. Steffen, R. K. Johnson, D. Reader, A. H. Lichtenstein, Physical Activity American Heart Association Nutrition Committee of the Council on Nutrition, Council on Arteriosclerosis Thrombosis Metabolism, Council on Cardiovascular Disease in the Young Vascular Biology, and D. the American. "Nonnutritive Sweeteners: Current Use and Health Perspectives: A Scientific Statement from the American Heart Association and the American Diabetes Association." *Circulation* 126, no. 4 (2012): 509–519.

Miller, P. E., and V. Perez. "Low-Calorie Sweeteners and Body Weight and Composition: A Meta-Analysis of Randomized Controlled Trials and Prospective Cohort Studies." *The American Journal of Clinical Nutrition* 100, no. 3 (2014): 765–777.

Thomas, O., L. Thabane, J. Douketis, R. Chu, A. O. Westfall, and D. B. Allison. "Industry Funding and the Reporting Quality of Large Long-Term Weight Loss Trials." *International Journal of Obesity* 32, no. 10 (2008): 1531–1536.

Lyn O'Brien Nabors retired as president of the Calorie Control Council in 2011, having worked with the Council for over

30 years. Ms. Nabors is the editor of four editions of Alternative Sweeteners, *a comprehensive textbook providing fundamental scientific and technical information on a broad range of sweeteners. She also has authored a number of book chapters and numerous journal articles on low-calorie foods and beverages, sweeteners, and fat replacers. She currently consults for the food industry.*

Shape Up America! Vision for the Future: Focus on Childhood Obesity and Parenting

Barbara J. Moore

When Shape Up America! was founded 20 years ago, obesity was widely considered to be a vanity issue, best not discussed. But data published in well-regarded medical journals showed that obesity was vying with smoking as the leading cause of preventable death in the United States. This finding commanded the attention of C. Everett Koop, MD, Sc.D., who had served as the 13th U.S. Surgeon General, and was viewed as the "nation's doctor" well after he had left that office in 1989.

Five years later, Dr. Koop founded Shape Up America! with the mission to raise awareness of obesity as a health issue rather than a cosmetic issue. Well before any other public health leader, Dr. Koop spoke out about the threat of obesity to health, social and emotional well-being and called upon the media, educators, policymakers, employers, and health care professionals to contribute to efforts to stem the growing prevalence of obesity. Yet, since that time, we have watched the data on obesity prevalence sharply increase in people from all walks of life and in all age and ethnicity categories. Only in recent years has the growing epidemic of obesity showed signs of slowing.

In 2014, the *New England Journal of Medicine* published a large longitudinal study of children who were followed from kindergarten through to eighth grade. The majority of children who were obese when they entered kindergarten remained obese through eighth grade. Approximately half of the overweight kindergarteners became obese by the time they reached eighth grade. This study strongly suggests that intervention during infancy and early childhood to prevent the development of obesity in toddlers and preschoolers should become a top priority.

Yet, to prevent the development of obesity in preschoolers, intervention during pregnancy or even prior to conception may well be necessary. The rigid concept that our genes are our destiny is slowly being replaced by a more sophisticated and nuanced understanding of the process by which phenotype is expressed. Our genetic inheritance may explain a predisposition for obesity, but over the next 10 years I expect scientists to develop a clearer understanding of the mechanisms by which other factors, such as diet, exercise, and specific nutrients, can influence the very shape of our genes, and thereby influence genetic expression. This is the domain of epigenetics—a relatively new field of science that will yield startling new insights into the etiology of obesity.

I fully expect that new findings in the field of epigenetics will inform the evidence base for the prevention of childhood obesity. It will be our responsibility, as translators of science and educators, to clearly communicate these new findings to all sectors of the public, taking care to delineate the behavioral factors such as diet and exercise, parental engagement, and feeding practices that influence genetic expression.

It is not widely appreciated that the single most powerful predictor of childhood obesity is obesity in biological parents—both paternal as well as maternal obesity—although the contribution of the latter appears to be somewhat stronger, possibly because of the female's role in pregnancy. Furthermore, studies show that the more severe the level of obesity in parents, the higher is the risk in the offspring. Genetic and epigenetic research should be focused on the biological mechanisms explaining the linkage between parental obesity and offspring obesity. I expect that research will provide future generations with a better understanding of how environmental and cultural factors either strengthen or weaken the linkage.

The influence of obesity on oogenesis, spermatogenesis, conception (including assistive reproductive technology), implantation, and fetal development will also be a focus of research attention. Hopefully, these findings will lead to changes in the educational curriculum for preteens and teens, so that they graduate from high school with a better understanding of energy balance and how the choices they make as youth will influence their own epigenetic endowment and the many controllable factors that influence the health and development of their offspring.

As a culture, we do little to prepare young people to be good parents. Yet skilled parenting plays an important role in the prevention of childhood obesity. We need to do more to teach young people about the growth and development of infants and children, provide them with basic cooking skills, fundamental principles of food and nutrition, and other important parenting knowledge and skills. A shift to a culture of health will certainly recognize the importance of sound parenting skills and how important they are for shaping brain development, taste preferences, and appetite regulation in children.

As our understanding of the importance of parenting continues to grow, I would expect that public policies and programs would be well established that are grounded in an improved scientific understanding of factors that protect against childhood obesity. My vision for the future is to have all children graduate from high school with a clear understanding of energy balance. Our educational system must equip students with the knowledge and skills needed to maintain a healthy diet and physically active lifestyle, navigate and improve our obesogenic environment, and above all to nurture and raise healthy children.

Barbara J. Moore, Ph.D. has extensive experience in development of obesity-related programs and policy. Dr. Moore is currently president and chief executive officer of Shape Up America! She was recruited for Shape Up America! in 1995 by former U.S. Surgeon General Dr. C. Everett Koop. In 2003, the Institute of Medicine of the National Academy of Sciences in Washington D.C. appointed Dr. Moore to serve on its committee to develop an "Action Plan to Prevent Obesity in Children and Youth." This was her second appointment by the Institute of Medicine, having served from 2001 to 2003 on a subcommittee to research and report on the growing problem of weight management in the U.S. armed forces.

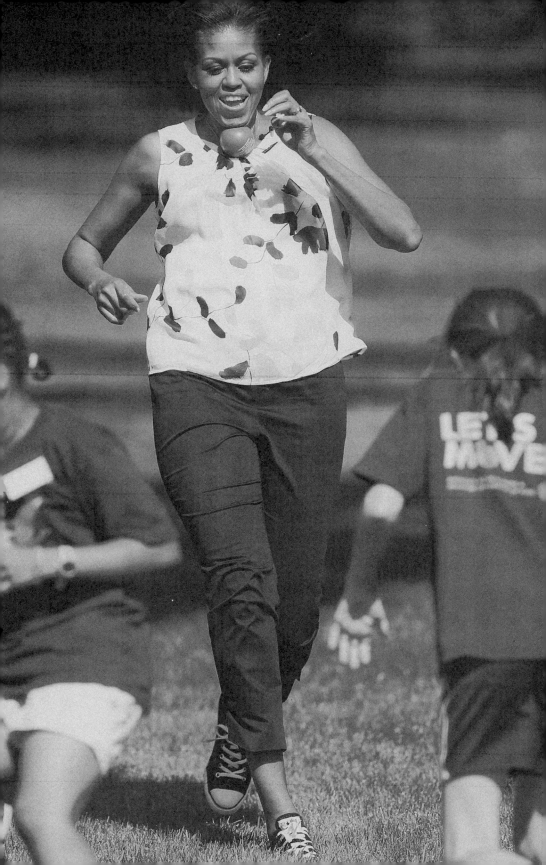

4   Profiles

One way of understanding more about obesity is by learning about the lives and work of individuals and organizations who have been involved in that subject. This chapter provides brief biographical sketches of a number of important men and women in the field as well as organizational sketches of involved groups. The profiles included here are only a sample of the untold number of individuals and organizations involved in this field over the past half century or more.

Activists, Thinkers, and Researchers

S. Daniel Abraham (b. 1924)

S. Daniel Abraham, born and raised in Long Beach, New York (1924), served as an infantryman in the U.S. Army during World War II. After the war, he bought the Thompson Medical Company. In the late 1950s, his first diet product was Slim-mint gum, which contained benzocaine and was supposed to decrease hunger. This was followed in 1976 by Dexatrim, which contained phenylpropanolamine (PPA) and was a one-a-day weight loss pill. It was reformulated when PPA was linked to an increased risk of strokes. The "new" Dexatrim

Health professionals, activists, and organizations are committed to raising obesity awareness and to improving access to its prevention and treatment. At the national level, Michelle Obama, wife of the 44th president of the United States, created the Let's Move! campaign that supports schools, families, and communities in fostering environments that encourage healthy choices that could prevent childhood obesity. (AP Photo/Carolyn Kaster)

contained ephedrine, which was linked to adverse health effects, and Dexatrim was reformulated again.

According to Forbes, in the late 1970s, he "shook up the weight-loss industry with his Slim-Fast nutrition drinks." It made losing weight simple. He sold the company to Unilever for $2.3 billion (2000). The title of his memoirs (2010) is *Everything Is Possible: Life and Business Lessons from a Self-Made Billionaire and the Founder of Slim Fast.*

David Allison (b. 1963)

David Allison, born in New York City (1963), has a B.A. (Vassar College, 1985) and a Ph.D. (Hofstra University, 1990). His two postdoctoral fellowships were at Johns Hopkins School of Medicine and Columbia University's N.Y. Obesity Research Center (1991–1994). He joined the faculty as assistant professor of Psychology (1994) and was promoted to associate professor (1999) Columbia University College of Physicians and Surgeons. He joined the faculty of the University of Alabama at Birmingham (2001) where he is professor of Biostatistics, head of the Section on Statistical Genetics, and director of an NIH-funded Clinical Nutrition Research Center.

His research casts a wide net (obesity, quantitative genetics, clinical trials, statistical and research methodology, research integrity). Dr. Allison is known for his work on the relations among obesity, weight loss, mortality or longevity, and his work on the genetic and environmental influences on obesity. He challenges conventional ideas, explores novel hypotheses, and holds himself and others to rigorous standards of evidence. He has authored over 300 scientific papers and edited five books. He is a Fellow of the American Statistical Association (2007), the Society for Design and Process Science (2004), and Institute of Medicine (National Academies, 2010). Awards include: Lilly Scientific Achievement Award (The Obesity Society, 2002), Andre Mayer Award (International Association for the Study of Obesity, 2002), Presidential Award for Excellence in Science, Mathematics and Engineering Mentoring (2006). He met with President George W. Bush in the Oval Office.

Elizabeth Applegate (b. 1956)

Elizabeth Applegate was born in 1956 in a nuns' convent near Johannesburg, South Africa, where her father was doing uranium ore research. She obtained her Ph.D. from the Department of Nutrition at University of California at Davis (1983) where she is senior lecture and director of Sports Nutrition for Intercollegiate Athletics. Her undergraduate nutrition course is the largest in the nation (more than 2,500 annually). Her 25-year nutrition column *Fridge Wisdom* in *Runner's World* is easy to read and understand. Dr. Applegate has authored several books, including *Encyclopedia of Sports and Fitness Nutrition* (2002), *Nutrition Basics for Better Health Nutrition* (2011), and *Eat Smart Play Hard* (2001). She has appeared in TV shows such as The CBS Early Show, Good Morning American, CNN, ESPN, and the Discovery Channel, and is often quoted in national print media like the *LA Times*, *Washington Post*, and *USA Today*. Dr. Applegate's research includes the effects of natural food products on exercise performance.

Arne Astrup (b. 1955)

Arne Astrup was born in Frederiksberg, Denmark (1955). He obtained his M.D. (1981) and Sc.D. (1986) from the Faculty of Health Sciences, University of Copenhagen. Dr. Astrup is professor and head of the Department of Human Nutrition at The Royal Veterinary and Agriculture University (Copenhagen, Denmark). He is known for his research on metabolism in the etiology and treatment of obesity. Some of his research investigates a new hormone, adiponectin, secreted by adipose tissue. It is involved in insulin sensitivity (improves it) and development of atherosclerosis (decreases the risk). Weight loss increases plasma adiponectin. A low-calorie diet improved glycemic control in overweight patients with type 2 diabetes.

Dr. Astrup, internationally known for his leadership, was president of the International Association for the Study of Obesity (2006–2010) and is editor-in-chief of *Obesity Reviews* (1999–). Some of his awards include: Knight of the Order of

Danneborg (1999), Servier Award for Outstanding Obesity Research (1999), and IASO Andre Mayer Award (1994).

Robert C. Atkins (1930–2003)

Robert C. Atkins was born in Columbus, Ohio (1930). He has a B.A. (University of Michigan, 1951) and M.D. (Cornell Medical College, 1955). He was a physician, cardiologist, and founder of the Atkins Center for Complimentary Medicine. In a 2003 interview by Larry King on CNN, Atkins was introduced as being "the world's most controversial diet guru."

Dr. Atkins is best known for his controversial popular diet that was very low in carbohydrates and high in protein and fat. You can eat steak, eggs, and cheese but not chocolate. His first diet book, *Dr. Atkins' Diet Revolution: The High Calorie Way to Stay Thin Forever* was published in 1972. The Atkins Diet Plan has been modified to include more carbohydrates, which are gradually introduced after about a week where they severely restrict refined carbohydrates to less than 50 calories daily or about one tablespoon of sugar. His books have been number one on the New York Times best-seller lists. His last book was *Atkins for Life: The Complete Controlled Carb Program for Permanent Weight Loss and Good Health* (2003).

A number of celebrities have been on the Atkins diet, including Julia Roberts, Catherine Zeta-Jones, Brad Pitt, and Al Gore. Stevie Nicks, of Fleetwood Mac, called him "a God among men." Atkins died in 2003 from injuries after he slipped on ice.

Richard L. Atkinson (b. 1942)

Richard L. Atkinson was born in Petersburg, Virginia (1942). He graduated from Virginia Military Institute (1964) and received his M.D. from the Medical College of Virginia (1968). He was a faculty member at the University of Virginia (1977–1983), University of California at Davis (1983–1987), Eastern Virginia Medical School (1987–1993), and the University of

Wisconsin where he is emeritus professor of Medicine and Nutritional Sciences.

Dr. Atkinson is known for his pioneering research in virus-induced obesity. Atkinson and his colleague, Dr. Nikhil Dhurandhar, demonstrated that a human adenovirus (Ad-36) produced obesity in animals and was associated with obesity in humans. Their research was not initially accepted by the scientific community; it was dismissed and heavily criticized. Today, their research is viewed as an important breakthrough that may help to explain our worldwide obesity epidemic. Dr. Atkinson also did some of the early research on intestinal bypass surgery on obese rats.

Dr. Atkinson is editor of the *International Journal of Obesity* (2000–). He is clinical professor of pathology at Virginia Commonwealth University and director of the Obetach Obesity Research Center. Drs. Atkinson and Judith S. Stern were cofounders of the American Obesity Association (1995), a lay advocacy organization which is now part of The Obesity Society. Atkinson and Stern were the first recipients (2006) of The Atkinson-Stern Award for Distinguished Public Service awarded annually by The Obesity Society.

George Blackburn (b. 1936)

George Blackburn was born in McPherson, Kansas (1936). He received his M.D. from the University of Kansas (1965), and did his internship and residency at Boston City Hospital, Harvard Medical School. He obtained his Ph.D. in nutritional biochemistry from Massachusetts Institute of Technology (1973). He is a general surgeon and fellow of the American College of Surgery and pioneered the development of Roux-en-bypass.

Dr. Blackburn is the S. Daniel Abraham associate professor of Surgery and Nutrition, associate director of the Nutrition Division (Harvard Medical School), and director of the Center for Nutrition Medicine (Beth Israel Deaconess Medical Center). He is committed to expanding research and treatment for obesity and nutrition. Dr. Blackburn was the past president of The Obesity Society, American Society for Clinical Nutrition, and American Society of Parenteral Nutrition. He was a board member of the American Obesity Association and is a Scientific Advisory Committee member of Shape Up America! Dr. Blackburn cochairs the Reality Coalition—an organization aiming to spread the message for healthy, moderate weight loss.

Dr. Blackburn has published over 400 papers. He is on the editorial board and a reviewer for journals such as *Journal of the American Medical Association, New England Journal of Medicine, American Journal of Clinical Nutrition*, and *Obesity*. Some of his honors include: Grace Goldsmith Award (American College of Nutrition 1988) and Goldberger Award in Clinical Nutrition (American Medical Association, 1998). He is an honorary member of the American Dietetic Association (1992).

Steven N. Blair (b. 1939)

Steven N. Blair was born in Mankato, Kansas (1939). He has a B.A. (Kansas Wesleyan University, 1962) in physical education and an M.S. and P.E.D. (Indiana University, 1965, 1968). He became PE instructor at the University of South Carolina (1966) and progressed through the ranks to professor. He worked at the Dallas-based Cooper Institute for 22 years where he was a researcher, director of research, and ultimately president and CEO (1980–2002). Dr. Blair returned to the University of South Carolina (2006) as professor in the Arnold School of Public Health.

Dr. Blair studies the associations between lifestyle and health, with a specific emphasis on exercise, physical fitness, body composition, and chronic disease. American seniors, who get a regular dose of physical activity, live longer than unfit adults, regardless of their body fat. This finding was based on his 12-year Aerobics Center Longitudinal Study. He has published over 410 papers and chapters, and was senior scientific editor for the U.S. Surgeon General's Report on Physical Activity and Health.

Some of Dr. Blair's awards and honors include: honorary doctorates (Free University of Brussels, Lander University, University of Bristol), Surgeon General's Medallion (1996), Honor Awards (American College of Sports Medicine), Fellow (American Epidemiology Society, American Heart Association, American College of Sports Medicine, The Obesity Society), Person of the Year for International Racket Sports Association (1990), and *Runner's World* All Star Team (1985). His work has been cited more than 44,000 times.

Claude Bouchard (b. 1939)

Claude Bouchard was born in Quebec, Canada (1939). He has a bachelors (Laval University, 1962), masters (University of Oregon, 1963), and doctorate (University of Texas, Austin, 1977). He held the Donald Brown Research Chair on Obesity (Laval University, 1997–1999). In 1999, he became executive director of the Pennington Biomedical Research Center in Baton Rouge, one of the world's leading nutrition and preventive medicine research centers.

Dr. Bouchard has done extensive research on genetics and a predisposed link of some people to obesity. His most influential work is the response of identical twins to long-term overfeeding. The twins were overfed 84,000 calories over 12 weeks. They gained almost 15.5 lbs. Some twins were low gainers and others were high gainers, but individual pairs of twins gained a similar amount of weight.

Dr. Bouchard has written several books and over 800 scientific papers. He was president of The Obesity Society (1991–1992) and International Association for the Study of Obesity (2002–2006) and a member of the Board of the American Obesity Association. Honors include: Honor Awards (Canadian Association of Sport Sciences, 1988), American College of Sports Medicine Citation (1992), honorary doctorate

(Katholieke Universiteit Leuven 1998), Royal Academy of Medicine of Belgium (member, 1996), and TOPS Award (The Obesity Society).

George A. Bray (b. 1931)

George A. Bray was born in Evanston, Illinois, in 1931. He has a B.A. (Brown University, 1953) and an M.D. (Harvard Medical School, 1957). Dr. Bray is a leader in promoting the concept that obesity is a disease and not the result of gluttony, sloth, and moral issues.

Dr. Bray's academic appointments were at the Tufts University, Harbor-UCLA Medical Center, University of Southern California, and Louisiana State University. He was the first executive director of the Pennington Biomedical Research Center, Baton Rouge (1989–1998), where he is currently Boyd professor and professor emeriti of medicine (Louisiana State University).

Dr. Bray's contributions to the field of obesity are impressive. He is internally recognized for his research in obesity and diabetes, and has published over 1,500 scientific papers, reviews, books, and abstracts. He cofounded and was president of The Obesity Society and editor of three journals (*International Journal of Obesity, Obesity,* and *Endocrine Practice*). He was president of International Association for the Study of Obesity and American Society for Clinical Nutrition, board member of The American Obesity Association, and a member of the Advisory Council of the National Institute of Diabetes, Digestive and Kidney Diseases. He is a member of Weight Watchers Scientific Advisory Board (2014). Dr. Bray has an interest in the history of medicine. While editor of *Obesity Research*, he wrote a series of 36 historical essays that have been collected in a book called *The Battle of the Bulge* (2007).

His many honors include: the Bristol-Myers/Squibb Mead Johnson Award in Nutrition, Fellow of American Association for the Advancement of Science, Osborne-Mendel and

McCollum Awards (American Nutrition Society), Goldberger Award in Nutrition (American Medical Association), Take off Pounds Sensibly and Stunkard Lifetime Awards (The Obesity Society), Willendorf Award (International Association for the Study of Obesity), and honorary membership in the American Dietetics Association. The Obesity Society gives a George Bray Founder's Award.

Kelly Brownell (b. 1951)

Kelly Brownell was born in Evansville, Indiana (1951). He has a B.A. in psychology (Purdue University, 1973) and a Ph.D. in clinical psychology (Rutgers University, 1977), and did an internship at Brown University. He joined the faculty in the Department of Psychiatry at the University of Pennsylvania (1977). He moved to Yale University as professor (2000) where he was professor of Psychology, Epidemiology and Public Health, and director of the Rudd Center for Food Policy and Obesity. He is currently dean of the Sanford Center of Public Policy at Duke University (2013).

Dr. Brownell is internationally known for his expertise on eating disorders and obesity. One of his famous early studies was conducted in a shopping mall, train station, and a bus terminal in Philadelphia, Pennsylvania, where stairs and escalators were adjacent. He placed a simple, colorful sign that said, "Your Heart Needs Exercise, Here's Your Chance." The number of people using the stairs increased. Fewer obese people took the stairs. When the sign was removed, stairs use decreased and escalator use increased.

Dr. Brownell coined the phrase "toxic environment," which applies to many factors which have contributed to obesity. These include food marketing directed at children, large portion sizes, foods in schools, economic imbalance where healthy foods costs more than unhealthy foods, lobbying strength of food and agribusiness companies, and failure to harness the law in the service of improving nutrition. One of his books,

Food Fight, details these environmental drivers of obesity and proposes a number of possible policy solutions (paperback edition, 2010). Dr. Brownell and colleagues did pioneering studies on "weight cycling" and coined the phrase "yo-yo dieting," to describe the cycles of weight loss and regain experienced by so many dieters. He has written 14 books and published more than 300 scientific papers and articles. He consults with members of Congress, appears often on television, and is frequently quoted in newspapers and magazines. In 2006, he was named by *Time* magazine as one of the World's 100 Most Influential People. He was elected to the Institute of Medicine in 2010.

Henry Buckwald (b. 1932)

Henry Buckwald was born in Vienna, Austria, in 1932. He came to America with his family to escape the Nazis during World War II. He received his M.D. from Columbia University (1957). He served in the U.S. Air Force as a captain and flight surgeon (1958–1960). He then attended University of Minnesota and received an M.S. in biochemistry and a Ph.D. in surgery. He is professor in the Department of Surgery at the University of Minnesota and was holder of the Davidson Wangensteen Chair in Experimental Surgery.

Dr. Buckwald is known for his work in bariatric surgery, especially with respect to its co-morbid outcomes. He has helped to improve both the type of operations done and the overall quality of bariatric surgeons. One of his seminal research studies, published over 40 years ago, demonstrated that even before there is weight loss, bariatric surgery improves insulin resistance and decreases the "bad" cholesterol.

Dr. Buckwald was president of three organizations (Central Surgical Association, American Society for Bariatric Surgery, and International Federation for the Surgery of Obesity). He is head of the Obesity Coalition, a national organization that includes most of major academic groups in the United States. One of its missions involves obesity management. He is chair of the American College of Surgeons National Faculty for Bariatric Surgery (2003–). Dr. Buckwald received Inventor of the Year Award and inducted into the Minnesota Hall of Fame (1988) for establishing the field of metabolic surgery, which later evolved to bariatric surgery.

Jenny Craig (b. 1932)

Jenny Craig was born Genevieve Guidroz in Berwick, Louisiana (1932), and raised in New Orleans. She worked for Nutrisystems (a weight loss company). Jenny and her husband Sid moved to Australia for two years, where she started The Jenny Craig Weight Loss Program (1983) because there was no comprehensive weight loss program in Australia. She knows what it is to be obese, having gained 50 lbs with the birth of her second daughter. Jenny Craig, Inc. has weight loss centers in the United States, Canada, Puerto Rico, and New Zealand. In 2002, the couple sold the majority of their interests in Jenny Craig, Inc (2002) to a New York and London-based private investment firm ACI Capital.

Nikhil Dhurandhar (b. 1960)

Nikhil Dhurandhar was born in 1960 in India where he obtained his M.D. As a physician and nutritional biochemist, he has been involved in obesity treatment for over 25 years and has treated over 10,000 patients using lifestyle therapy and pharmacological approaches.

Dr. Dhurandar started his research with the adenovirus (AD 36) in India. He continued this research at the University of Wisconsin with Dr. Richard L. Atkinson, and then at the Pennington Biomedical Research Center in Baton Rouge.

Dr. Dhurandhar and his colleagues were the first to show an association between adenoviruses and obesity in people. Dhurandhar and Dr. Richard L. Atkinson looked for the presence of antibodies in people. More obese people had antibodies than lean people. This research was not initially accepted by the scientific community—in fact, it was dismissed and heavily criticized. Today, this research is viewed as an important breakthrough that may help to partially explain our worldwide obesity epidemic.

Dr. Dhurandar is professor and chair of the Department of Nutritional Sciences at Texas Tech University in Lubbock, Texas (2014–). His research continues to focus on the role of adenoviruses in causing obesity and the potential for developing a vaccine to obesity. His honors include: the Osborne Mendel Award (American Society for Nutrition, 2015). He is president of The Obesity Society (2014–2015) and editor of the *International Journal of Obesity*.

William H. Dietz

William Dietz has a B.A. (Wesleyan University, 1966), M.D. (University of Pennsylvania, 1970), and a Ph.D. (Massachusetts Institute of Technology, 1981). He is director of the Strategies to Overcome and Prevent (STOP) Obesity Alliance (2014) at the Milken Institute of Public Health (George Washington University). He is a pediatrician and one of the first researchers to pay attention to the issues surrounding overweight in children. For example, he was first to demonstrate a relationship between television viewing and obesity. He has published over 150 papers and is editor of four books.

He was professor of Pediatrics at Tufts University School of Medicine and director of Clinical Nutrition at the Floating Hospital of New England Medical Center Hospitals until 1997, when he became director of the Federal Center for Disease Control in Atlanta, Georgia (1997–2012). He has helped support states to develop and evaluate strategies to prevent obesity. This approach is based, in part, on Dietz's research, which indicated that there was something going on during adolescence that makes a person more susceptible to the complications of obesity as an adult. He has been instrumental in reclassifying children who are currently called "at risk of overweight" to "overweight." This has been criticized by those who believe that this may wrongly classify many children as "diseased," in spite of the fact that the BMI cutoff points for overweight and obesity are arbitrary and not precise.

Some of his honors include: election to the Institute of Medicine of the National Academy of Sciences (1998), past president of the American Society of Clinical Nutrition and The Obesity Society, honorary member of the American Dietetic Association (2002), recipient of John Stalker Award (American School of Food Service Association, 1995), and the Bray Founders Award (The Obesity Society, 2005).

Adam Drewnowski (b. 1948)

Adam Drewnowski was born in Warsaw, Poland (1948). He has a B.A. (Oxford University, 1971) and Ph.D. (The Rockefeller University, 1978). After his postdoctoral training (University of Toronto), he returned to The Rockefeller University as an assistant professor. He then moved to the University of Michigan as professor of public health, psychology and psychiatry and director of the program in Human Nutrition. In 1998, he joined the faculty at the University of Washington in Seattle where he is director of the Nutritional Science Program and director of the Center for Public Health Nutrition and UW Center for obesity research.

Dr. Drewnowski is internationally known for his research in taste, food preferences, and obesity. His research focuses on the relationships between poverty and obesity, and links between diabetes and obesity rates in vulnerable populations, and access to healthy foods.

Johanna Dwyer (b. 1938)

Johanna Dwyer was born in Syracuse, New York (1938). She has a B.S. (Cornell University, 1960), M.S. (University of Wisconsin, 1962) and a M.S. and Sc.D. (Harvard University School of Public Health, 1969). After several years on the faculty of

HSPH, she moved to Tufts University where she is professor of Medicine and Community Health (School of Medicine and Freidman School of Science Nutrition and Public Policy). Her government service includes: assistant administration for Human Nutrition (USDA 2001–2002) and senior nutritionist (Office of Dietary Supplement at NIH, 2003).

Dr. Dwyer was a member of the U.S. Dietary Guidelines Committee (2000) and the Food and Nutrition Board of the National Academy of Sciences (1992–2001). Her honors include: election to IOM (2000), Atwater Award (American Society of Nutrition, 2005), Elvejhem Award (ASN, 2005), Distinguished Alumnae Award (HSPH 2004), and past president of the American Society of Nutrition and Society for Nutrition Education. She is the editor of *Nutrition Today*.

Dr. Dwyer's career has been devoted to expanding the scientific basis for clinical and public health interventions, especially in obesity and cardiovascular disease. She has written and published over 475 scientific articles.

Katherine M. Flegal (b. 1944)

Katherine M. Flegal was born in 1944 in Berkeley, California. She has a Ph.D. in nutritional sciences (Cornell University, 1982) and completed a postdoctoral fellowship in epidemiology (University of Pittsburgh, 1984). She was a research faculty member (University of Michigan University of Michigan, 1984–1987) prior to joining the National Center for Health Statistics (CDC, 1987–). She is also an adjunct professor at the University of North Carolina School of Public Health.

Dr. Flegal is internationally known for her research in the epidemiology of obesity. She tracks changing prevalences and epidemiologic trends of overweight in children and adults in the United States. Using data from the National Health and Nutrition Examination Survey (NHANES), she reported that people who are overweight (BMI 25.0–29.9), but not obese, have a lower risk of death from heart disease and cancer than those of normal weight. The figure of deaths associated with obesity was 112,000 rather than the 365,000 used by the American Medical Association (*Journal of the American Medical Association*, 2005). In a subsequent paper (2007), Dr. Flegal reported that overweight (BMI more than 25) was associated with increased mortality from diabetes, cardiovascular disease, and certain cancers, but not other causes of death.

Dr. Flegal is a member of numerous professional organizations and advisory committees. Some of these include: associate editor (*American Journal of Epidemiology*), Advisory Committee Endocrinologic and Metabolic Drugs (FDA), Committee on Statistics (American Heart Association), Center for Alaska Native Health Research (University of Alaska, Fairbanks), and Center for Weight and Health (University of California, Berkeley).

Jared Fogle (b. 1977)

Jared Fogle was born in Indianapolis, Indiana (1977). He was featured in an advertising campaign for Subway (the national chain that specializes in selling submarine sandwiches). When he was a junior in high school, he weighed 425 lbs and wore work size 6XL shirts. He blamed the start of his weight problems to "the best birthday present of my life"—a Nintendo. He used a one-hand approach and had the controller in one hand and a bag of chips in the other.

Jared developed his own "Subway Diet" by eating a 6-inch turkey sub for lunch and a 12-inch sub, chips, and a diet coke for dinner. After 3 months, he lost almost 100 lbs. By the end of his diet, he lost about 250 pounds. A former dorm mate wrote an article about Jared's weight loss experience. A reporter for *Men's Health* magazine included *The Subway Diet* in an article entitled "Crazy Diets that Work." He was "discovered" by the creative director at Subway's advertising agency, and they started a regional ad campaign. The first spot aired in January 2000. The commercial had a disclaimer: "The Subway diet, combined with a lot of walking, worked for Jared. We're not saying this is for everyone." The campaign went "national" and he has toured the country for Subway with his "fat pants." By 2013, he had filmed more than 300 commercials and continues to make appearances and speeches for the company. Subway attributes one-third to one-half of its growth in sales to Fogle.

Jeffrey M. Friedman (b. 1954)

Jeffrey Friedman was born in 1954 in Orlando, Florida. "Growing up was just like any other suburban place—a zillion kids on bicycles and playing sports constantly." His has a B.S. in biology (Renssalaer Polytechnic Institute) and an M.D. (Albany Medical College of Union University in a combined 6-year program, 1977). He did two residences (Albany Medical Center Hospital and Cornell University). Dr. Friedman has a Ph.D. in molecular biology (The Rockefeller University, 1986). He joined the faculty at The Rockefeller University as an assistant professor (1986) where he is the Marilyn Simpson professor and head of the Laboratory of Molecular Genetics.

One of Dr. Friedman's publications in the journal *Science* was an essay "A War on Obesity, Not the Obese." It subsequently was included in the *Best American Science and Nature Writing 2004* anthology (Houghton Mifflin). Interestingly, the first paper he wrote was rejected with the comment, "This paper should not be accepted at the *Journal of Clinical Investigation*—or anywhere else."

Dr. Friedman's codiscovery of the hormone leptin (1994) and its role in regulating body weight have changed our understanding of the causes of human obesity. Some of his honors include: election to the Institute of Medicine (2005), Distinguished Achievement in Metabolic Research (Bristol-Myer, 2001), Passando Foundation Award (2005), the Gairdner Foundation International Award (2005).

M. R. C. Greenwood (b. 1943)

Mary Rita Cooke Greenwood was born in 1943 in Gainesville, Florida. She has a B.A. (Vassar College, 1968) and a Ph.D.

(The Rockefeller University, 1973). She joined the faculty at the Institute of Human Nutrition at Columbia University (1969–1978). She returned to Vassar College (1978) and became department chair and John Guy Professor of Natural Sciences (1986–1989). Dr. Greenwood moved to the University of California at Davis as dean of Graduate Studies (1989–1993), and then became Chancellor of University of California at Santa Cruz (1996–2004). She was senior vice president and provost at the University of California (2004–2005). She returned to UC Davis (2005–2009) where she was distinguished professor and director of the Foods for Health Program. She was president of the University of Hawaii (2009–2013). She is distinguished professor emeritus at the University of California at Davis.

Dr. Greenwood has played a leadership role in obesity research and policy. She made significant contributions to the way we do science as associate director for Science at the Office of Science, Technology and Policy during the Clinton Administration (1993–1995). She is one of the cofounders of The Obesity Society and past president (1987–1988). Her honors are numerous and include: election to Institute of Medicine (1992), fellow, past president, and chair of the Board of Directors of the American Association for the Advancement of Sciences, member of the American Academy of Arts and Sciences, and recipient of the American Presidential Citation Psychological Association (1995).

Barbara Hansen (b. 1941)

Barbara Hansen was born in Boston, Massachusetts (1941). She has a B.S. (University of California, Los Angeles) and a Ph.D. (University of Washington, Seattle). Dr. Hansen is currently professor of Internal Medicine and Pediatrics and director of both the Centers for Preclinical Research and Obesity, Diabetes, and Aging Research at the University of Tampa, Florida. She has also been director of the Obesity, Diabetes and

Aging Research Center and vice president for graduate Studies and Research (University of Maryland, Baltimore).

Dr. Hansen is internationally known for her research in obesity, diabetes, and aging. She has over 200 scientific publications. Her classic work in monkeys demonstrated that prevention of obesity by maintaining their weight when they were young adults reduced the risk for the development of type 2 diabetes in middle and old age. Her research has significantly added to the body of knowledge that humans and nonhuman primates have an extraordinary ability to regulate appetite, body weight, and body composition. This system is influenced by age-related changes and has a very strong genetic basis.

Some of the honors include: membership in Institute of Medicine (1981), Bray Founder's Award (The Obesity Society), McCollum Award (American Society for Clinical Nutrition—ASCN), McCollum Award (American Society of Nutritional Sciences), and president of the following societies: The Obesity Society, International Association for the Study of Obesity, and the ASCN.

Marion M. Hetherington (b. 1961)

Marion Hetherington was born in Helensburgh, Scotland (1961). She obtained a bachelor's degree in Psychology (University of Glasgow, 1982), trained as a teacher at Jordanhill College of Education (1983), and received her doctorate in Experimental Psychology (University of Oxford, 1987). She received a Fulbright Scholarship (1987) and worked with Dr. Barbara J. Rolls at Johns Hopkins University School of Medicine. She was awarded a Fogarty International Fellowship to do research at the National Institutes of Health (1988–1990). She was department chair in Psychology at University of Liverpool (2001–2004). Dr. Hetherington is the Caledonian Futures Professorship in Biopsychology at Glasgow Caledonian University (2005–). She was president of the Society for the Study of Ingestive Behavior (2009). Dr. Hetherington serves on the Association for the Study of Obesity committee and on the editorial board of the *British Journal of Nutrition*.

Dr. Hetherington is known for her work on short-term influences on food intake, including sensory-specific satiety. She has published extensively with Dr. Barbara J. Rolls. Hetherington also investigated gene–environment interactions in the development of obesity. Her current research focuses on early determinants of overeating in children. She has studied the impact of school-based healthy eating interventions in areas of material deprivation in Glasgow.

James O. Hill (b. 1951)

James O. Hill was born in Crossville, Tennessee (1951). He has a B.S. (University of Tennessee) and a Ph.D. (University of New Hampshire). He is professor of Pediatrics and Medicine at the University of Colorado at Denver. Dr. Hill was chair of the WHO Consultation on Obesity (1997), president of The Obesity Society and American Society of Nutrition (2008), and is a vice president of the International Association for the Study of Obesity. He was a member of the Expert Panel that developed the National Institutes of Health Guidelines for Management of Overweight and Obesity and was chair of the first World Health Organization Consultation on Obesity.

He established the programs "Colorado on the Move" (2002) and "America on the Move" (2003), which are national health initiatives to help tackle the obesity epidemic and inspire Americans to aim for healthier lifestyles. He believes that the "small changes" approach to lifestyle modification is the best way to reverse the obesity epidemic. Along with Dr. Rena Wing, he is also known for his stewardship of a "National Weight Control Registry," which follows over 6,000 people who have lost weight and kept it off permanently. He has spent over 25 years researching the causes of weight gain, adiposity, and obesity, and how to prevent or treat these problems. Dr. Hill's research interests are how diet and physical activity affect body weight and how they are connected to the obesity epidemic. His work with families showed that small changes in diet and physical activity can be achieved and sustained and call help family members avoid excessive weight gain. He has published over 300 scientific articles and lectures widely about weight management. Dr. Hill wrote *The Step Diet Book* to help people both lose weight and keep it off.

Hippocrates (460 BC–370 BC)

Hippocrates was born in 460 BC on the Greek island of Kos. He was the founder of the Hippocratic School of medicine and is known as the father of western medicine. Hippocrates was thousands of years ahead of his time when he said that it was very injurious to health to take in more food than the constitution will bear, when at the same time one uses no exercise to carry off this excess. He warned his fellow Greeks that sudden death is more common in those who are naturally fat than in the lean.

Jules Hirsch (b. 1927–2015)

Jules Hirsch was born in New York City (1927). He is one of few physicians that went to medical school (University of Texas, Austin, 1948) without a college degree. He joined the faculty at The Rockefeller University where he is professor emeritus and physician-in-chief emeritus. Some of his honors include: election IOM (1993) and the 2006 recipient of an award from The Obesity Society.

Dr. Hirsch is unofficially known as "Dr. Fat Cell." His classical research found that obese people can have more fat cells, large fat cells, or a combination of the two in comparison with people who are not obese. Weight loss decreased the size of fat cells but not the number. He showed that different fat depots can respond differently to hormones and other compounds. Hirsch has also done research in psychology. He reported that people, who are obese since childhood, if they lose weight as adults, continue to "see" themselves as fatter than they really are. He fed a small number of subjects different liquid formulas containing equal calories, but as high in fat or high in carbohydrates. Weight loss was not changed when subjects switched formulas. He has trained and worked with a number of leaders in obesity, including M.R.C Greenwood, Judith S. Stern, Rudolph Leibel, and Patricia R Johnson.

W.P.T. James (b. 1938)

W.P.T. James was born in 1938 in Liverpool, England. He has a bachelor's degree from University of London (1959), a medical degree from UCH, London, and a Sc.D. (1983). He was appointed to the London School of Hygiene and Tropical Medicine (2008).

Dr. James is literally an international ambassador whose travels have highlighted the growing problem of childhood obesity in developing countries. He is founder and head of the International Obesity Task Force (IOTF; 1996), which is part of the International Association for the Study of Obesity, and chair of the World Health Organization (WHO) Presidential Council of the Global Prevention Alliance. IOTF is demanding action to deal with the childhood obesity crisis. He is responsible for the WHO classification of BMI for obesity. In the United States, this lowered the point at which adults are considered overweight from a BMI of 27–25.

His honors include: fellow of both the Royal College of Physicians in London and Edinburgh, Commander of the British Empire for Services to Sciences, Honorary Doctor of Science (City University of London), and founding member of the U.K. Academy of Medical Sciences. He was director (1982–1999) of the Rowett Research Institute in Aberdeen, which made substantial contributions to health and agricultural development around the world.

Patricia R. Johnson (b. 1931)

Patricia R Johnson was born in 1931 in Waco, Texas. She has a B.A. and M.A. (Baylor University, 1952, 1956) and a Ph.D.

(Rutgers University, 1967). She was a faculty member at Vassar College (1964–1989), chair of the Department of Biology (9 years), and Associate Dean of the College (4 years). She joined the Department of Nutrition at University of California, Davis (UCD) as research professor in 1990. She is currently emeritus from both Vassar College and UCD.

Dr. Johnson was responsible for the establishment and use of the genetically obese Zucker rat in the laboratory. Compared to lean rats, obese rats had extremely large and greatly increased numbers of fat cells. Weight loss decreased the size but not the number. Decreasing food intake did not decrease obesity. She did similar studies on obese mice. This represented a major advance in how we now view obesity. Dr. M. R. C. Greenwood collaborated with her on some of these studies.

Robin B. Kanarek (b. 1946)

Robin Kanarek was born in Pittsburgh, Pennsylvania (1946). She has a B.A. (Antioch College, 1963) and Ph.D. in psychology (Rutgers University, 1974). She was a postdoctoral fellow (Department Nutrition, Harvard University School of Public Health, 1974–1976) and a research fellow (School of Medicine, UCLA, 1979–1980). Since 1976, Dr. Kanarek is at Tufts University where she was chair of the Psychology Department, dean of the School of Arts and Sciences, and the John Wade professor of Psychology.

Dr. Kanarek's research focuses on the role of diet and exercise in determining behavioral consequences of neuropeptides related to food intake and on the effects of refined carbohydrates on the development of obesity and diabetes. She demonstrated that, in addition to leading to obesity and its related metabolic deficits, intake of highly refined carbohydrates, like sugar, can result in impairments in cognitive behavior. Dr. Kanarek is co-author or editor of three books and over 100 book chapters and papers. She was a member of the Institute of Medicine's Committee on Military Nutrition Research, associate editor of *Nutritional Neuroscience*, on the editorial boards of *Physiology and Behavior* and the *Tufts Diet and Nutrition Newsletter*, and past editor-in-chief of *Nutrition and Behavior*.

Janet King (b. 1941)

Janet C. King was born in Red Oak, Iowa (1941). She received a B.A. (Iowa State University, 1963). After completing a dietetic internship at Walter Reed General Hospital (1964), she worked at Fitzsimons Hospital in Denver, Colorado. A rotation in the Nutrition Research Lab exposed her to the excitement of human nutrition research. She has a Ph.D. in human nutrition (University of California at Berkeley, 1972) and was immediately appointed to its faculty in the Department of Nutritional Sciences (1972–1995) where she served as chair of the Department and Graduate Program. Dr. King directed the USDA Western Human Nutrition Research Center (1995–2003). She is a senior scientist at Children's Hospital Oakland Research Center (2003) and holds professorial appointments at UC Berkeley and UC Davis.

Dr. King is internationally known for her studies of the effect of maternal nutrition and the metabolic adjustments of pregnancy. She is studying effects of different diets on hormonal and metabolic pathways linked to poor pregnancy outcomes in obese women.

Dr. King served on numerous national and international committees, including chair of the Institute of Medicine (IOM) Food and Nutrition Board and Committee on Gestational Weight Gain, member of Dietary Guidelines Advisory Committee. Some of her many honors include: Institute of Medicine member (1994), USDA Agricultural Research Service Hall of Fame (2007), Fellow of the American Society for Nutrition (ASN; 2007), and Elvehejm Research Award (ASN; 2007).

Ahmed Kissebah (1937–2013)

Ahmed Kissebah was born in 1937 in Dumiat City, Egypt. Some of his advanced degrees include an M.D. (Cairo University, 1961) and a Ph.D. in molecular biology (University of

London, 1973). He joined the faculty at the Medical College of Wisconsin in Milwaukee (1977) where he was professor of Medicine and director of The TOPS Obesity and Medical Research Center.

Dr. Kissebah published over 200 papers. His research interests included body fat distribution, metabolic syndrome, and examining how genetics and obesity are related. His most significant contribution is the recognition that the distribution of body fat has an impact on the risk for obesity-related diseases. For example, obese women with excess fat, mainly around the waist, chest, neck, and arms (upper body obesity or apple shape), are at greater risk for developing type 2 diabetes than those with excess fat mainly about the thighs and buttocks (pear shape). He used circumference of the waist and the hip to estimate body fat distribution. He calculated the waist-to-hip ratio (WHR). In women, lower body obesity was a WHR of less than 0.76 and upper body obesity was a WHR of more than 0.85. This revolutionary work is a benchmark for many novel ideas in obesity research. He was also part of an international team of scientist that discovered that a gene on chromosome 15 regulates inflammation. This finding has had major implications for obesity.

Dr. Kissebah was medical director of Take off Pounds Sensibly (TOPS). TOPS members volunteered for his studies, allowing him to study genetics of obesity in families over three plus generations. He authored the book *The Choice Is Yours: A Practical Guide to Take Off and Keep off Pounds Sensibly*.

Some of his honors included: Outstanding Foreign Investigator (Japan), Distinguished Armour Award (President of Egypt), Princess Margaret Distinguished Research Award (Great Britain), and the King Faisel Distinguished Scientist Award (Saudi Arabia).

C. Everett Koop (1916–2013)

C. Everett Koop was born in Brooklyn, New York (1916). He has a B.A. (Dartmouth, 1937), an M.D. (Cornell Medical College, 1941), and Sc.D. (University of Pennsylvania, 1947).

Dr. Koop spent the majority of his career as a pediatrician at Children's Hospital of Philadelphia where he was surgeon-in-chief. He was professor of surgery at Dartmouth Medical School and senior scholar of the C. Everett Koop Institute.

He was best known for starting the practice of placing warning labels on packs of cigarettes when he was surgeon general of the United States (1982–1989). He said that had he stayed surgeon general longer, he would have tackled obesity.

In 1994, Dr. Koop founded Shape Up America!, a nonprofit national initiative, which has raised the awareness of health eating and increased physical activity for obesity prevention and disease management. He has many honors, including 35 honorary doctorates, Legion of Honor Medal (France, 1980), Public Health Distinguished Service Medal, and Institute of Medicine member (1989). Dr. Koop also won an Emmy (1991) for a television series on health care reform.

John Kral (b. 1939)

John Kral was born in 1939 in Sweden. He received his M.A. in Education and Behavioral Neuroscience (1961), M.D. (1967), and Ph.D. (1976) from the University Goteborg, Sweden. Dr. Kral was recruited to St. Lukes Hospital Center at Columbia University in New York City. He came to State University of New York Downstate Medical Center (1988) as professor of Surgery and Medicine and director of Surgical Services in the Department of Surgery.

Dr. Kral established a program of surgical treatment of obesity with a strong research component. His current research is in pediatric obesity and investigating its relationships to maternal stress in the inner-city environment. He has published more than 50 chapters and reviews and 60 peer-reviewed papers in high impact journals. Dr. Kral is a pioneer in bariatric surgery and one of the cofounders of the American Society for Bariatric Surgery (1983).

Shiriki Kumanyika (b. 1945)

Shiriki Kumanyika was born in Baltimore, Maryland (1945). She has a B.A. (Syracuse University, 1965), M.S. in social work (Columbia University, 1969), and a Ph.D. in Human Nutrition (Cornell University, 1978). She is professor in the Department of Biostatistics and Epidemiology at the University of Pennsylvania's School of Medicine.

Dr. Kumanyika has been engaged in obesity research since the mid-1980s. She has more than 250 publications. She founded and chairs the African American Collaborative Obesity Research Network. This reflects her strong commitment to reducing obesity and related health disparities in African American communities and to increasing the engagement of African American scholars in obesity research. Dr. Kumanyika has served on numerous advisory or expert panels and workgroups related to nutrition and obesity research and policy for NIH, IOM, WHO, and IASO. Some of her honors include: Bolton Corson Nutrition Research Medal (Franklin Institute, 1997), Population Research Prize (American Heart Association, 2005), *American Journal of Health Promotion*'s Symbol of H.O.P.E. (Award *American Journal of Health*, 2006), and IOM member (2003).

Jack LaLanne (1914–2011)

Jack LaLane was born Francois Henri LaLanne in San Francisco (1914). He attended Oakland Chiropractic College in San Francisco. He is known as "the godfather of physical fitness." In the 1930s, LaLane invented the Smith Machine, a barbell that was on steel runners and could only move up and down, which is used for weight training. He opened the first modern health spa in the United States in 1946. In 1951, he brought exercise to TV. His show was on TV for 34 years. It was the longest running TV show that was devoted to fitness. He encouraged women to lift weights, even though it was thought that it would make women unattractive.

Jack LaLanne was ahead of the "whole food movement" when he used to say "If man made it, don't eat it." When asked what he thought about organic foods, LaLanne replied "It's a bunch of bull. If you want to eat more organic that's fine, but I don't go out of my way to get to organic vegetables." When he was 70, he was handcuffed and shackled and swam 1.5 miles towing 70 boats with 70 people from the Queen's Way Bridge in the Long Beach Harbor to the Queen Mary. At 97 years old, Jack LaLane was inducted into the California Hall of Fame (2008) by California first lady, Maria Shriver. His mission was "To help people help themselves, feel better, look better, and live longer."

Antoine Lavoisier (1743–1794)

Antoine Lavoisier was born in Paris in 1743. During his brief lifetime, he studied chemistry, botany, astronomy, and mathematics at the College of Mazarin (1754–1761) and law at University of Paris (1761–1763). He is known as the father of modern chemistry. He was elected into the Royal Academy of Science (1768).

While working for the French government, he helped develop the metric system of weights and measures. He is best known for his discovery of the role that oxygen plays in combustion. Using a calorimeter, designed by Pierre Laplace (a French physicist and mathematician), he demonstrated that burning involves the combination of a substance with oxygen. He conducted experiments that demonstrated that respiration was a slow combustion of organic material using inhaled oxygen. This research forms the basis for measuring calories in food.

Unfortunately, Lavoisier used the results of others without acknowledging them. For example, Lavoisier tried to take credit for the work of Joseph Priestley, who discovered that when hydrogen combines with oxygen the result is water.

Lavoisier was tried as a traitor, convicted, and guillotined on May 8, 1794, by the French Revolutionists. Lavoisier's importance to science can be summarized by the quote of one of his colleagues: "It took them only an instant to cut off his head, but France may not produce another like it in a century."

Rudolph Leibel (b. 1942)

Dr. Leibel has a B.A. (Colgate University, 1963) and an M.D. (Albert Einstein College of Medicine, 1967). He was an intern and junior resident in pediatrics (Massachusetts General Hospital, 1967–1969) and then served in the U.S. Army Medical Corps (1969–1971). He is the Christopher J. Murphy professor of Diabetes Research, professor of Pediatrics and Medicine, and director of the Division of Molecular Genetics at Columbia University Medical Center (New York City).

He has been steadfast in his belief that "body weight was the result of complex interactions between genes and the environment rather than a matter of free will."

His honors are numerous and include: Institute of Medicine member (1998), Berthold Medal of the European Society of Endocrinology (2008), TOPS Scientific Achievement Award (The Obesity Society, 1996), Federation of Medical Scientific Societies of the Netherlands, Leiden University (2008), and honorary doctorate (Louisiana State University/Pennington Biomedical Research Center). Dr. Leibel has coauthored over 300 scientific papers, which have been cited over 13,000 times. He has been on numerous news shows and is often quoted in the popular press. Dr. Leibel was a key scientific commentator on HBO's *The Weight of the Nation* Series (2012).

Maimonides (1135–1204)

Maimonides (Moses Ben Maimon) was born in Cordoba, Spain (1135). He was thought to be the greatest physician of his time. He treated luminaries like the Sultan Saladin and Richard the Lionheart. He wrote many medical texts. Some of these texts have survived and have been translated into English. Some of his comments about obesity still apply to the 21st century:

Obesity is harmful to the body and makes it sluggish . . . Extremely obese individuals should travel to the seashore, do much walking in the sun, and bathe in the sea in order to lose weight . . . Their nutrition should consist of foods that are not very nourishing such as vegetables, (especially) onions and garlic . . . things which strengthen without (adding) moisture, such as roasted meat from non-fat meats. (The obese). . . should drink little and should perform as much (physical exercise). . . as possible. (*The Medical Aphorisms of Moses Maimonides*, translated by Fred Rosner and Suessman Muntner. Bloch Publishing, 1973. Vol 1, p 193 [treatise 9, #101]).

Jean Mayer (1920–1993)

Jean Mayer was born in Paris, France (1920). He was the son of Andre Meyer, a famous French physiologist. He was a professor at the Harvard University School of Public Health and became president and chancellor of Tufts University. He was an advisor to three presidents (Nixon, Ford, Carter) and had a column in the *Boston Globe*.

Dr. Meyer was internationally known for his research in obesity and for the discovery of how hunger is regulated by the amount of glucose in the blood (i.e., glucostatic hypothesis). In a 1973 *Time* magazine article about McDonald's, Dr. Mayer was quoted that "the menu provides large amounts of fats and calories (557 for a Big Mac, 317 in a chocolate shake, 215 for a small order of fries), and contains almost no roughage. There is nothing at McDonald's that makes it necessary to have teeth."

Barbara J. Moore (b. 1947)

Barbara J. Moore was born in Paterson, New Jersey (1947). She has a Ph.D. (Columbia University, 1983). Her post-doctoral training was taken at the University of California Davis. She was an assistant professor at Rutgers University (1987–1989).

Dr. Moore has extensive experience in development of programs and policy at both the private and public level. She left academia and became general manager of Program Development for Weight Watchers International (1989–1993). She spent two years in Washington, D.C., at the National Institutes of Health and the White House Office of Science and Technology Policy. She was recruited in 1995 by former U.S. Surgeon General Dr. C. Everett Koop for his newly founded Shape Up America! (SUA!) initiative. At SUA!, she raised the awareness of obesity as a health issue and has developed responsible information on weight management for the media, educators, health care professionals, and the policy makers.

Jean Neiditch (1923–2015)

Jean Neiditch was born in Brooklyn, New York (1923). She started the original Weight Watchers in the early 1960s. She invited friends weekly to her home in Queens, New York City. They exchanged information about how to lose weight. This enterprise grew into Weight Watchers International, a successful business with about a million members worldwide attending 400,000 groups each week.

Michelle Obama (b. 1964)

Michelle Obama was born in Chicago (1964). She addresses obesity through promoting good eating habits and physical activity (*Let's Move*). She is the wife of the 44th president of the United States (Barack Obama). Her legacy will be in the area of childhood obesity. She created the Task Force on Childhood Obesity to review current programs to create a national plan for change.

Xavier Pi-Sunyer (b. 1933)

Xavier Pi-Sunyer was born in Barcelona, Spain (1933). He has a B.A. (Oberlin College, 1955), M.D. (Columbia College of Physicians and Surgeons, 1959), and an M.P.H. (Harvard

University School of Public Health, 1963). He is currently professor of Medicine at Columbia University, director of the VanItallie Center for Weight Loss and Maintenance, and chief of the Division of Endocrinology, Diabetes, and Nutrition.

Dr. Pi-Sunyer's extensive research interests include lipid and carbohydrate metabolism, obesity, and diabetes. He has developed a model to study fat, proteins, and bone mineral changes with weight loss in pre- and postmenopausal women. He has published over 250 scientific papers and numerous review articles and book chapters. Some of his honors include: fellow (American Heart Association), Stunkard Lifetime Career Award (The Obesity Society, 2000), Bray Founders Award (The Obesity Society, 2006), Luken Medal and Lecturer (American Diabetes Association, 1977), and two honorary doctorates (University Rome, University Barcelona).

Dr. Pi-Sunyer was president of the American Diabetes Association, American Society for Clinical Nutrition, and The Obesity Society. He was chairman of the Task Force on Treatment of Obesity (NIH) and member of the board of directors for Weight Watchers Foundation. He chaired the controversial NIH panel that reclassified many normal weight Americans as "overweight" (1998).

Nathan Pritikin (1915–1985)

Nathan Pritikin was born in Chicago, Illinois (1915). He was a student at the University of Chicago from 1933–1935, but he did not get a degree. He was diagnosed with heart disease when he was only 41. He disobeyed his doctor's advice to keep on eating a diet of butter, ice cream and steaks. He put together his own diet high in unrefined carbohydrates and very, very low in fat. His blood cholesterol decreased from a high of 280 to a low of 120. He no longer had heart disease. In 1976, he founded the Pritikin Longevity Center, which today offers controlled diet, counseling in lifestyle change, and exercise in a spa/resort setting.

Barbara J. Rolls (b. 1945)

Dr. Barbara Rolls, born in Washington, D.C., in 1945, obtained a B.A. (University of Pennsylvania, 1966), an M.A. (University of Oxford, England, 1970), and a Ph.D. (University of Cambridge, England, 1970). She held several research fellowships at the University of Oxford (1969–1984). She joined the Johns Hopkins University School of Medicine faculty as associate professor of Psychiatry and Behavioral Sciences (1984) and was promoted to professor (1992). In 1992, she moved to Pennsylvania State University where she is professor of Nutritional Sciences and Behavioral Health and holds the Guthrie chair in Nutrition.

Dr. Rolls was past president of both the Society for the Study of Ingestive Behavior and The Obesity Society. Some of her numerous awards include: Human Nutrition Award (American Society of Nutritional Sciences), MERIT Award (NIH), International Award for Modern Nutrition, and Honorary Membership (American Dietetic Association), fellow of the American Association of the Advancement of Science (2006), Atwater Lecturer at Experimental Biology (EB), and Centrum Center for Nutrition Science Award (EB, 2008).

She is the author of over 200 original research articles on eating disorders, food preferences, and the effects of preloads of food on subsequent food intake. One of her papers found that increased portion sizes increase energy intake in a number of settings, including restaurants. The order in which you eat food can affect calorie intake. Eating large portions of hot soup at the start of a meal decreases food intake in the rest of the meal. She has written five books, including *Thirst, The Volumetrics Weight-Control Plan: Feel Full on Fewer Calories* (#5 on the *New York Times Bestseller*, 2007), and *The Volumetrics Eating Plan* (#1 on the *New York Times Bestseller*, 2007). Volumetrics is based on healthy strategies to enhance satiety. It has been widely used in weight loss clinics and was incorporated into the Jenny Craig Program.

Wim H. M. Saris (b. 1949)

Wim H. M. Saris was born in Zwolle, The Netherlands (1949). He has degrees in Human Nutrition (Wageningen University, 1974) an M.D. (1979), and Ph.D. (1982), both from the Catholic University of Nijmegen. He was appointed associate professor (1982) at Medical and Health Science Faculty at the Maastricht University where he is professor in Human Nutrition (1987–). In 1992, Dr. Saris initiated the Nutrition and Toxicology Research Institute (NUTRIM), a collaborative program. He was the first scientific director (1992–2005). In 2005, he became a part-time corporate scientist for human nutrition for the DSM Company at the Food Ingredients site in Delft.

Dr. Saris' obesity research is the experimental and public health aspect of obesity. He has written 7 books and over 350 scientific papers. He is on the editorial board of several scientific journals and national and international committees (e.g., Scientific Committee on Food of the European Commission and European Technology Platform initiative "Food for Life"). He was president of Netherlands Association of the Study of Obesity and European Pediatric Exercise Society. He coordinates the European Union (EU) sixth framework research project DiOGenes (Diet, Obesity, and Genes), the largest EU-funded obesity-related research program with 33 partners.

Ethan Allen Sims (1916–2010)

Ethan Allen Sims, born in Newport, Rhode Island (1916), has a B.A. (Harvard College, 1938), M.D. (Columbia College of Physicians & Surgeons, 1942), and was house officer and later instructor at Yale-New Haven Hospital (1946). Dr. Sims spent his entire academic career at the University of Vermont (1950) where he was professor of Medicine, emeritus.

His Vermont study of experimental weight gain opened new ways about thinking about obesity. To explain the relationship between obesity and diabetes, he coined the word *diabesity*.

This describes the result of genes interacting with other genes and environmental factors to produce obesity-induced type 2 diabetes. He asked the question: "What would happen if thin people who never had a weight problem deliberately got fat?" His subjects, prisoners at a state prison, volunteered to gain weight. For over 4–6 months, they increased their weight by 20–25 percent. Some had to consume 10,000 calories a day. He was featured in an April 16, 2002, article in the *New York Times* entitled "Is Obesity a Disease or Just a Symptom?" Honors include: Ethan Sims Clinical Research Feasibility Fund Award (NIH) and the Ethan Sims Young Investigator Award (The Obesity Society).

Sachiko St. Jeor (b. 1941)

Satchiko St. Jeor was born in Los Angeles, California (1941). She received her Ph.D. in nutrition (Pennsylvania State University, 1980) and is a registered dietitian. She is currently professor emeritus of Internal Medicine at the University of Nevada School of Medicine in Reno where she was professor and chief, Division of Medical Nutrition and director of the Center for Nutrition.

Dr. St. Jeor's research has focused on metabolism. The Harris-Benedict equation, developed in 1900, predicted the metabolic rate for men and women based on their age, weight, and height. With the changes in lifestyles since 1900, Drs. Mifflin and St. Jeor developed a new equation (Mifflin-St. Jeor) that is 5 percent more accurate and is being recommended for use today. She also developed methods for research diets used on metabolic wards and dietary intake analysis programs.

Dr. St. Jeor has been a member of many national committees, including 1995 Dietary Guidelines, "Weighing the Options" (IOM), Healthy Weight Roundtable (NIH), and Calcium Consensus Panel (AHA). Some of her honors include: Medallion Award and the Award for Excellence in the Practice of Dietetic Research (American Dietetic Association), fellow

(American Dietetic Association, AHA, Society of Behavioral Medicine), and the Marjorie Hulsizer Coper Award (2013), which is the highest award given by the Academy of Nutrition and Dietetics.

Albert J. Stunkard (1922–2014)

Albert J. Stunkard (Mickey) was born in Manhattan in 1922. He obtained his M.D. from Columbia University (1945). He was professor of Psychiatry emeritus at the University of Pennsylvania School of Medicine.

Dr. Stunkard was a pioneer in the studies of eating behavior. He was first to describe "binge eating" and develop a treatment. He was also first to describe "night eating syndrome" (NES; *Psychiatric Quarterly*, 1959), a new eating disorder linked to obesity. NES is associated with not being hungry in the morning, being hungry in the evening, and insomnia where people wake up frequently during the night and eat.

Dr. Stunkard did a large-scale study of the growth and development of children at high risk of obesity. These children have been studied since 3 months of age for over 10 years. The mothers are either lean or obese. Some of his important findings are related to food intake and body weight during the first year of life. These include the importance of sucking behavior at 3 months in predicting body weight and adiposity five years later, and the importance of rate of food intake in determining adiposity in subjects at high risk of obesity.

Two of Dr. Stunkard's many honors included member of Institute of Medicine (1988) and the creation of the Stunkard Lifetime Achievement Award (The Obesity Society, 2003) to recognize individuals who have made outstanding contributions to the field of obesity.

Oprah Winfrey (b. 1954)

Oprah Winfrey was born in 1954 in Kosciusko, Mississippi, in abject poverty. She studied speech and the performing arts at the Tennessee State University. She got a job in radio while in high school and coanchored the local evening news when she was 19, where she was the first black women to hold that job.

She is the American multiple-Emmy award winning host of the Oprah Winfrey Show, the highest-rated talk show in TV history. She has been called the "ultimate media icon." CNN has called her the "world's most powerful woman." *Vanity Fair* magazine has written that she has had "more influence on the culture than any university president, politician, or religious leader, except perhaps the Pope."

Winfrey has gone public with how difficult it is to lose weight. Oprah is one of the wealthiest people in the United States. She has a personal trainer (Bob Greene) and a chef. She has said that if there was a pill or a diet that magically caused weight loss, she would have it.

Rena Wing (b. 1945)

Rena Wing was born in New York (1945). She has a B.A. (Connecticut College, 1967) and a masters and doctorate ((Harvard University, 1971). Dr. Wing spent almost 25 years at the University of Pittsburg before moving to Brown Medical School (1998). Currently, she is professor of Psychiatry and Human Behavior and director of the Weight Control and Diabetes Research Center at the Miriam Hospital.

Dr. Wing is internationally known for her research on behavioral treatment of obesity and its application to type 2 diabetes. She was responsible for designing and overseeing the lifestyle intervention that was used in the Diabetes Prevention Program and was effective in reducing the risk of developing diabetes. Dr. Wing is chair of Look AHEAD, a NIH-funded study examining whether weight loss reduces cardiovascular morbidity or mortality in overweight individuals with type 2 diabetes. Dr. Wing developed the National Weight Control Registry (NWCR) with Dr. James Hill (1994). The NWCR includes over 5,000 individuals who have been successful in losing weight and maintaining it, and is important in increasing understanding of long-term weight loss maintenance.

Dr. Wing is known for her leadership in obesity and diabetes. She was a member of the NIH Task Force on Prevention and Treatment of Obesity, the Council of the National Institute of Diabetes, Digestive and Kidney Diseases, and president of the Society of Behavioral Medicine. She has published more than 250 peer-reviewed articles in the area of obesity treatment and prevention. Her honors include: the TOPS Award for outstanding achievement (The Obesity Society, 2001), the Dean's Teaching Excellence Award (Brown Medical School, 2003, 2005), and the Distinguished Contributions Award (Behavioral Medicine and Psychology Council of the American Diabetes Association).

David A. York (b. 1945)

David A. York was born in England in 1945. He received his B.S. and Ph.D. from the University of Southampton, England. He conducted postdoctoral research at the Medical Center Hospital in Boston, Massachusetts, and the UCLA School of Medicine. He moved back to Southampton University Medical School, where he was on the faculty for 18 years. He joined the Pennington Biomedical Research Center in Baton Rouge as the chief and subsequently associate executive director for Basic Research and the head of the Experimental Obesity Research Group. He was also a Boyd professor in the Louisiana State University System (1998–2005). He then became director for the Center for Advanced Nutrition at Utah State University (2006). He retired in 2014 and is currently adjunct professor at Wayne State University School of Medicine.

Dr. York has published more than 240 peer-reviewed papers. Some of his research interests include using animal models of obesity to study mechanisms that control food intake, nutrient selection, hormone dependence of animal obesity, and the molecular basis for the beneficial effects of exercise in preventing neurodegenerative disorders. He has presented or chaired at more than 100 major conferences. He was president of The Obesity Society (1999–2000), an Executive Committee Member/Treasurer of the International Association for the Study of Obesity/World Obesity Federation (1998–2014), and now chairs the Publications Committee of the World Obesity Federation. He is editor of *Obesity Reviews*, which is published by World Obesity Federation (formerly the International Association for the Study of Obesity). *Obesity Reviews* deals with controversial topics in obesity and presents pros vs. cons articles as well as standard reviews. Some provocative questions that have been addressed were: Food industry friend or foe? Is food addictive? Will reducing sugar-sweetened beverages reduce obesity?

Dr. York believes that a top public health concern in today's environment is the development of obesity. Understanding the mechanism(s) and the reasons for individual differences in susceptibility will provide us the needed insight into the role of nutrition in health and disease. Dr. York is one of the few researchers who is able to study nutrition from the whole animal down to the individual genes or molecular events that enables the nutritional response. His experimental approaches range from genomic studies, cell culture, neurobiology, and animal feeding behavior. While today's environment in which we live is conducive to the development of obesity, a top public health concern, and other chronic diseases, understanding the mechanisms and the reasons for individual differences in susceptibility will provide us needed insight into the role of nutrition in health and disease.

Agencies, Programs, and Organizations

The following agencies, programs, and organizations provide information, publications, and funding opportunities to encourage achievement and maintenance of a healthy weight. Some of the information is adapted from Web sites of agencies, programs, and organizations listed below. Use common sense when accessing information. Does the organization have any special interest that might make them put a spin on the information? What is the source of funding? These questions should be asked of all Web sites, including those that are consumer oriented, from nonprofit organizations, industry, or the government. The organizations are listed according to whether they are: (1) Government Agents and National Programs and Initiatives; (2) International Agencies and Organizations; (3) Non Profit, Professional and Trade Organizations.

Government Agencies and National Programs and Initiatives

Agricultural Research Service

The work of the Agriculture Research Services (ARSs) covers agriculture from field to table. It ensures that American agricultural products are safe, of good quality, and competitive within the world economy. ARS developed a number of high-fiber low-calorie products used by food companies as fat substitutes. Oatrim, for example, is used in products, such as frozen dinners and other products, to lower calorie and cholesterol content. Research on obesity prevention coordinates human nutrition with ARS crop studies, animal breeding, and new product and food-processing research. Research areas are based on learning what people eat, what the body needs, and how to modify foods to be more beneficial.

Centers for Disease Control and Prevention

The Centers for Disease Control and Prevention (CDC), under the Department of Health and Human Services (DHHS), tracks and investigates public health trends. It publishes weekly data on all deaths and diseases reported in the United States in the *Morbidity and Mortality Weekly Report*. It is a resource for fact sheets related to obesity prevention. The site provides an interactive body mass index calculator.

The Division of Nutrition, Physical Activity, and Obesity (DNPAO) within CDC helps prevent and control obesity by promoting regular physical activity and good nutrition. Activities include translating results of research into practical advice for medical professionals and the public. The *Research to Practice Series* discusses implications of newest studies on nutrition, physical activity, and obesity research. CDC worksites promote obesity prevention and control (e.g., demonstration projects at CDC worksites to adapt effective strategies into interactive Web-based tools for employers to design their own programs). Physical activity guidelines are developed in partnership with President's Council on Physical Fitness and Sports. The CDC collaborates with the WHO, a leader in building worldwide research, to study effective public health practices to combat obesity worldwide.

Center for Nutrition Policy and Promotion

The Center for Nutrition Policy and Promotion (CNPP), created in 1994, is an agency of the U.S. Department of Agriculture (USDA). It conducts research into consumer food behaviors (e.g., nutrition knowledge and attitudes, dietary survey methodology, nutrition education techniques). They also maintain estimates of overall nutrient content of the U.S. food supply since 1909. A staff of expert nutritionists, dietitians, economists, and policy experts link up-to-date scientific research with messages about healthful nutrition for Americans. CNPP publishes and publicizes the *Dietary Guidelines for Americans*, the basis for government nutrition policy and nutrition education activities. Guidelines are jointly reviewed and updated every five years by USDA and DHS. CNPP develops educational tools to put the Guidelines into practice (e.g., Food Guide Pyramid, MyPyramid for Kids, Steps to a Healthier Weight, MyPyramid PodCasts).

Department of Health and Human Services

Department of Health and Human Services (DHHS) aims to protect the health of Americans. Its 11 divisions administer over 300 programs. Besides publishing reports and guidelines, DHHS provides Web sites such as healthfinder.gov, which provides information on physical fitness, nutrition, and how to make healthy choices, along with interactive games to help children and teens learn about healthy eating and physical fitness.

Economic Research Service

Part of the U.S. Department of Agriculture (USDA), Economic Research Service (ERS) is the primary source of economic information and research about food and farming for policymakers and the public. One goal is to promote a healthy, well-nourished population. Data are used to study how obesity is affected by food supply and national eating patterns. ERS publishes consumer-friendly reports and *Amber Waves*, a magazine that contains in-depth feature articles, research findings, and previews of on-going research.

Food and Drug Administration

The Food and Drug Administration (FDA) is a federal regulatory agency within DHHS. It reviews toxicological research and clinical trials to approve or reject new drugs for the marketplace. The FDA Center for Food Safety and Applied Nutrition takes action against unsafe dietary supplements after they reach the market. It relies on consumers' reports of serious events through the MedWatch Program. One example was the case of ephedrine-containing weight loss products. Numerous adverse events were reported (chest pain, heart attacks, strokes, death). In 2004, FDA prohibited sales of dietary supplements containing ephedrine.

Its Web site has useful information for consumers and educators with links to topics, including dietary supplements, food labeling, nutrition, medical devices, drugs, and FDA program to combat obesity. A free electronic newsletter about dietary supplements contains information about ingredients used in weight loss products.

Food and Nutrition Service

The Food and Nutrition Service (FNS), a branch of USDA, provides families and children in need with easier access to nutritious foods through education and food assistance programs. It is responsible for National School Lunch, Food Stamp, and Women, Infant, and Children (WIC) food assistance programs. FNS recognizes that obesity is a serious health concern in America and their goal is to educate the public, especially children in school, to make healthy food choices.

National Heart, Lung, and Blood Institute

National Heart, Lung, and Blood Institute (NHLBI) is part of the National Institutes of Health. Its primary mission is to support basic and applied research related to heart, lung, and blood diseases. NHLBI established the Obesity Education Initiative (OEI) in 1991 to help decrease the incidence of CVD and type 2 diabetes by reducing prevalence of overweight and increasing physical activity. The OEI uses population-based and high-risk strategies. The population approach focuses on the general population with activities, which include promotion of physical education, a nutrition curriculum in schools, and Hearts N' Parks in partnership with the National Recreation and Park Association, to encourage increased daily physical activity. It targets individuals who are experiencing, or are at increased risk, for adverse health effects associated with overweight and obesity. An expert panel issued *Clinical Guidelines on the Identification, Evaluation, and Treatment of Overweight and Obesity in Adults: Evidence Report* (June 1998). These were the first federal clinical practice guidelines that analyzed overweight and obesity issues using an evidence-based approach and provided practical strategies for applying recommendations.

NHLBI has education activities for healthcare professionals and holds conferences for researchers at the NIH center. The Web site offers a wealth of information for the public, health professionals, and researchers, including latest health news, tools, tutorials, online slides, and an electronic textbook on obesity. NHLBI provides patient and public obesity treatment recommendations (*Aim for a Healthy Weight*).

National Institutes of Health

National Institutes of Health (NIH) is the chief Federal Agency responsible for conducting and supporting research with people. Studies range from small pilot projects to multi-center clinical trials and include lifestyle, pharmacological, and other medical approaches. Research focuses on diagnosis, prevention, treatment, and building a scientific evidence base for public policy decisions. A major NIH objective is to develop ways to explain research results from clinical trials to the medical community and the public. More than 80 percent of the $30 billion appropriated by Congress is used for funding research grants in the United States and some foreign countries.

The NIH Obesity Research Task Force published *Strategic Plan for NIH Obesity Research* (2004, updated in 2011), a multifaceted agenda for the study of behavioral and environmental causes of obesity with the study of genetic and biologic causes. The Plan detailed coordination of obesity research across NIH.

National Institute of Diabetes, Digestive, and Kidney Diseases

National Institute of Diabetes, Digestive, and Kidney Diseases (NIDDK) is one of the Institutes of NIH. It conducts and supports basic and clinical research on diabetes, digestive, and kidney diseases. It has an Office of Obesity Research because obesity is estimated to be a precipitating cause for 80 percent of type 2 diabetes and its complications. Weight Control and Healthy Living is one of the topics on the NIDDK Web site.

Office of the Surgeon General

The Office of the Surgeon General is part of DHHS. The surgeon general, appointed by the president, is a commissioned officer in the Public Health Service who holds the rank of a three-star vice admiral while in office. The surgeon general's role is to provide the best scientific information about how to improve our health and reduce risk of illness and injury. The Web site contains information on healthy eating and active living.

United States Department of Agriculture

USDA is the primary government agency for agriculture, food, and human nutrition. It has a number of divisions, including the Agricultural Research Service and Economic Research Service. One mission area is to improve health in the United States. For example, USDA's Center for Nutrition Policy and Promotion links scientific research to dietary guidance, nutrition policy coordination, and nutrition education. You can read the Dietary Guidelines for Americans Report and get information about physical activity and long-term weight loss. USDA's National Agricultural Library (NAL) is accessible online (http://www.nal.usda.gov) where you can view published research articles.

Weight-Control Information Network

Weight-Control Information Network (WIN), an information service of NIDDK at NIH, focuses on getting up-to-date, science-based information to the public and media about weight control. WIN covers the range from underweight, to normal weight, and to obesity. It provides information about risks associated with overweight/obesity with special emphasis on diabetes. WIN provides tip sheets, fact sheets, and brochures for a range of audiences.

International Agencies and Organizations

Food and Agricultural Organization of the United Nations

The Food and Agricultural Organization (FAO), a United Nations agency, has a major effort to reduce malnutrition and hunger. Obesity is not as big a problem as hunger; but obesity is rapidly increasing in developing nations. FAO's approach to preventing the problem from getting worse is through public education in every country. Its objectives are to promote good nutrition and physical activity, and agriculture policy that encourage consumption of healthy foods.

Health Canada

Health Canada is the national department responsible for helping Canadians achieve good health while respecting individual choices and circumstances. The Health Canada Office of Nutrition Policy and Promotion defines, promotes, and implements evidence-based nutrition policies and standards. The Web site provides information about health-related legislation and activities. There are links to other Canadian government sites that provide additional information about obesity.

International Federation for the Surgery of Obesity

International Federation for the Surgery of Obesity (IFSO) is an umbrella for 34 national associations of bariatric surgeons. Its goal is to bring together surgeons and allied health professionals (e.g., anesthesiologists, dietitians, internists, nurse practitioners, nutritionists, psychologists), who are involved in the treatment of very obese patients. The main goal is to optimize treatment of severely obese patients. The organization has a set of guidelines for selection criteria for patients and minimal requirements for bariatric surgeons. IFSO is committed to creating a system for accreditation for individual surgeons and bariatric centers around the world. The Web site contains information about treatments, scientific articles, and meetings. IFSO has a yearly World Congress which, along with the online forum, provides an opportunity for surgeons to exchange knowledge on surgical treatment of severely obese patients, to present new techniques, research and concepts, and to meet the experts in the field. The Web site has interactive movies about obesity such as causes, risks, and descriptions of bariatric surgical procedures. There are links to its publication *Obesity Surgery Journal* and a listing of bariatric surgeons.

International Obesity Task Force

International Obesity Task Force (IOTF) is the advocacy arm of IASO. It works with partners in the Global Prevention Alliance to support new strategies to improve diet and activity and prevent obesity. IOTF works with the WHO and other private and public groups. With a special emphasis on preventing childhood obesity, their goal is to alert people around the world about the urgency of the obesity problem and to persuade governments to act now. Publications and research news about a range of obesity-related issues can be accessed on the IOTF Web site. The site also presents useful links to government agencies, academic institutions, and resources for health-related information.

World Health Organization

WHO is the directing and coordinating authority for health within the United Nations. Its six general goals are promoting development, fostering health security, strengthening health systems, harnessing research, information, and evidence, improving performance, and enhancing partnerships. In the area of obesity, WHO sponsors the Commission on Ending Childhood Obesity. Its Web site provides a wealth of fascinating information about international health topics, programs, and projects, and interactive pages with data and statistics about obesity in individual countries.

Nonprofit, Professional, and Trade Organizations

American Academy of Family Physicians

American Academy of Family Physicians (AAFP), a national organization, represents 94,000 family physicians, family medicine residents, and medical students. It has a guide for family physicians to help their overweight patients and launched a

10-year fitness initiative called "Americans in Motion." AAFP asserts that there is ample evidence for recognizing both childhood overweight and adult obesity as a disease, and that insurance companies should reimburse family physicians that provide reasonable diagnosis and treatment of overweight and obesity. The Web site has a number of sections that have excellent information for families, including answers to common questions and weight issues for children. There are links to other sites (e.g., U.S. Department of Health and Human Services, Office of Disease Prevention and Health Promotion, Reuters Health) which also provide information about obesity. Its produces a semi-monthly, peer-reviewed journal entitled the *American Family Physician*.

Academy of Nutrition and Dietetics

The Academy of Nutrition and Diatetics (AND) is a professional organization of dietitians with expertise in nutrition, food, and health. It is the largest organization of food and nutrition professionals in the world, with more than 68,000 members. Dietitians play an important role helping people manage and prevent overweight and obesity by showing them how to formulate reasonable weight goals and personalized eating patterns that can be sustained over the long term. AND publishes *Journal of the American Dietetic Association* and position papers on health issues, including weight control. The Web site has a variety of information about food and nutrition, as well as a referral service that can link consumers with registered dietetic professionals.

American Academy of Pediatrics

The American Academy of Pediatrics (AAP) is a national professional association dedicated to the health of all infants, children, adolescents, and young adults. AAP was instrumental in developing medical policies and guidelines for childhood obesity as part of the important Expert Committee Recommendations

Regarding Prevention, Assessment, and Treatment of Child and Adolescents. *Pediatrics*, its peer-reviewed journal, has been published since 1948.

American Cancer Society

The American Cancer Society (ACS), a nonprofit organization funded by donations, is dedicated to helping patients, friends, and family learn more about cancer. Its Web site is extensive and informative. People can get help to make decisions about cancer treatment and finding treatment centers. There is a survivor network. ACS advocacy activities have influenced Congress, state governments, and have been instrumental in getting over $1 billion annually for the National Cancer Institute for research.

With respect to obesity, people who are overweight or obese are at increased risk for developing certain cancers. ACS presents research about the relationship between obesity and cancer. *Take Control of Your Weight* includes guidelines for weight loss and a chance to plan a healthful diet with a virtual dietitian. Many materials on the site have been translated into Spanish and several Asian languages.

American College of Physicians

The American College of Physicians (ACP) is a national organization of physicians who specialize in prevention, detection, and treatment of chronic illnesses such as diabetes and obesity. ACP, established in 1915, is a membership organization for physicians who treat adults. *Annals of Internal Medicine* is widely cited. On their Web site, there is a section for patients with information about obesity. The Internal Medicine Report gives access to published papers and videos about important medical and health issues.

American College of Preventive Medicine

The American College of Preventive Medicine (ACPM) is a national professional society for U.S. doctors with about 2,000 members. It focuses on disease prevention and health promotion in individuals and in population groups. Physicians trained in preventive medicine work in primary care, in public health and government agencies, in workplaces, and in academia. ACPM has an official Position Statement about optimal diet for weight control that discourages the use of fad diets. They publish the *American Journal of Preventive Medicine*; some of their articles are related to obesity.

American College of Sports Medicine

The American College of Sports Medicine (ACSM), a nonprofit organization, has 20,000 members with expertise in sports medicine, exercise physiology, physical activity, and cardiovascular health. ACSM collaborates with other organizations and issues consensus statements. These position statements are published in the College's scientific journal, *Medicine & Science in Sports & Exercise*. The ACSM Web site has a news release section which provides information about obesity and nutrition, including "Dispelling the Top 10 Nutrition Myths."

American Council on Science and Health

The American Council on Science and Health (ACSH) is a nonprofit, consumer education consortium primarily funded by industry. It has a Board of 350 physicians, scientists, and policy advisors. Experts review ACSH reports and participate in educational activities. ACSH is concerned with issues relating to food, nutrition, chemicals, pharmaceuticals, lifestyle, the environment, and health. Some publications include Health Effects of Obesity, Foods are not Cigarettes: Why Tobacco Lawsuits Are Not a Model for Obesity Lawsuits, and Childhood Obesity. The News Center Section of its Web site lists articles from ACSH that have been published in the popular press. You can get daily emails about current events.

American Diabetes Association

The American Diabetes Association (ADA) is a nonprofit health organization whose mission is to find ways to prevent, cure, and manage diabetes. It funds research, publishes scientific findings, provides information, and other services to people with diabetes. Both consumers and health professionals may become members. There is excellent information about obesity on its Web site. For example, there are sections on weight loss and exercise, recipes for healthy eating, research updates, and an easy-to-use body mass index calculator.

American Heart Association

The American Heart Association (AHA) is a nonprofit, national, voluntary health agency with professional and public members. The organization supports heart disease research, scientific meetings, and advocacy. It publishes several scientific journals and magazines for people concerned about prevention and treatment of heart disease. You can get a subscription to *Heart Insight*, a quarterly patient magazine that is free to people who live in the United States. On the Web site at HeartHub, there is a video on healthy eating, a body mass index calculator, tips on eating well, and losing weight. There are downloadable publications in both English and Spanish, such as *How can I manage my weight?* (*Respuestas del Corazon*) and *Losing Weight the Healthy Way* (*Controlando su peso*).

American Institute for Cancer Research

The American Institute for Cancer Research (AICR) encourages research on the relationship of nutrition, physical activity, and weight management to cancer risk, interprets the scientific literature, and educates the public about the results. It also supports health professionals with educational materials and advice in planning programs on diet, nutrition, and cancer prevention. AICR's second expert report, *Nutrition, Physical Activity, and the Prevention of Cancer: A Global Perspective*, confirmed the relationship between excess body fat and increased cancer risk. AICR experts stressed that many cancers are preventable. In fact, maintaining a healthy weight may be the single most important way to protect against cancer.

Information on its Web site changes often in response to popular news stories. One section *Ever Green, Ever Hungry* has articles about preventing winter weight gain, findings linking food, activity, and body weight to risk of colon cancer. Another one is "Eat to Satisfy your Body—Not to Satisfy Your Friends." You can subscribe to AICR's free e-newsletter.

American Medical Association

The American Medical Association (AMA), founded in 1847, is a membership organization of physicians. It publishes one of the most widely read medical journals, the *Journal of the American Medical Association*. Its Web site provides links to reports, publications, and resources about the health effects of overweight and obesity.

American Public Health Association

The American Public Health Association (APHA) has been working to improve public health since 1872. The Association's goal is to protect Americans from preventable health threats and to assure that health promotion, disease prevention, and preventive health services are accessible to everyone in the United States. It works with members of the Congress, regulatory agencies, and other public health organizations to influence policies and set priorities on a wide variety of issues that range from children's health, managed care, disease control, health disparities, bioterrorism, international health, and tobacco control. The APHA announced that preventing obesity in children is one of the most important public health issues facing the nation. It encourages development of new approaches and partnerships. In the *American Journal of Public Health*, aimed at public health workers and academics, special emphasis is given analysis of current public health issues in a historical context. The Web site provides tools and plans for individual and community efforts to tackle obesity.

American Society for Bariatric Surgery

The American Society for Bariatric Surgery (ASBS), founded in 1983, is a nonprofit medical organization made up of surgeons and other healthcare professionals. Its vision "is to improve public health and well being by lessening the burden of the disease of obesity and related diseases throughout the world." It publishes the scientific journal *Surgery for Obesity and Related Diseases*. ASBS offers educational programs for physicians, other healthcare professionals, and the public about bariatric surgery and guidelines for ethical patient selection and care. The society promotes outcome studies and measures of quality assurance to improve the safety and effectiveness of obesity surgeries. The Web site has information about extreme obesity, bariatric surgery, and diabetes.

American Society of Bariatric Physicians

The American Society of Bariatric Physicians (ASBP) is a national medical society of doctors offering medical treatment of obesity (bariatrics), weight loss, and dieting. There is a "Find a Clinician" section that lists contact information for bariatric physicians. There is no evaluation of the quality of the physicians. Its Web site contains up-to-date information and news about obesity treatment and medical weight loss.

Calorie Control Council

The Calorie Control Council (CCC) is a nonprofit organization supported by 60 companies that manufacture/sell low-calorie and reduced fat foods and beverages. The council provides understandable information about low-calorie sweeteners, like Aspartame, Saccharin, and Sucralose, and fat replacers, like Polydextrose and Olestra, for consumers interested in cutting dietary calories and fat. CCC has sponsored research on low-calorie ingredients, foods, and beverages, including studies about safety, metabolism, consumer use, and public opinion of food additives.

Center for Science in the Public Interest

Founded in 1971, the Center for Science in the Public Interest (CSPI) is an advocate for science-based information about nutrition and health, food safety, alcohol policy, and sound science. CSPI goals are to counter the food industry influence on public opinion and public policies and to lobby for government policies that are consistent with scientific evidence. CSPI also aims to educate the public. Its monthly newsletter, *Nutrition Action Health Letter*, has about 900,000 subscribers in the United States and Canada. It periodically reviews fad diets and issues about overweight and obesity. CSPI has been in the forefront of the efforts to require nutrition facts on packaged foods and to have calories of fast foods available at the point of purchase. It has also conducted studies on the nutrition quality of restaurant meals. CSPI works to improve food safety in an effort to decrease the number of food-borne illnesses. Its Web site has a section devoted to obesity.

The Clinton Foundation

The Clinton Foundation (TCF), in partnership with the American Heart Association, has created the Alliance for a Healthier Generation. Its mission is to eliminate childhood obesity in the United States and to encourage young people to develop lifelong healthy habits. To foster these changes that can make a difference to a child's health, the Alliance calls upon schools, industry, healthcare, the community, and children themselves.

The school programs focus on creating real, practical solutions to childhood weight management through healthier food choices and opportunities for activity in schools. The foundation created the *Healthy Schools Program* and *Kids Movement* to put healthy foods and beverages in vending machines and cafeterias, to increase opportunities for students to exercise and play at school, and to provide resources for teachers and staff to become healthy role models. Through the industry programs, TCF works with the food industry to persuade food purveyors, restaurants, and fast food outlets to produce healthier drinks, snacks, and meals that are available to children. It is also helping the healthcare industry to better understand, diagnose, and treat childhood obesity. The idea behind the *Kids Movement* plan was to motivate children to take charge of their health and to lead their own *Go Healthy* movement.

Consumers Union

Consumers Union (CU) is a nonprofit, independent testing and information organization. It publishes *Consumer Reports*. It does not accept advertisements so as to remain independent of bias. CU has reviewed weight loss supplements and diets and diet programs. Since many consumers log on to the Web for weight loss advice, *Consumer Reports* has rated dieting information sites and ranked the one that are most helpful. Some features or reviews are subscription only.

Council on Size and Weight Discrimination

The Council on Size and Weight Discrimination (CSWD) is a nonprofit group that is working to change attitudes about body weight on the job, in the media, and for medical treatment. Its Web site presents information and guidelines on how to become active in fighting weight discrimination.

Endocrine Society

The Endocrine Society, formed in 1916, supports research on hormones and the clinical practice of endocrinology. Worldwide, it has over 14,000 members who represent medicine, molecular and cellular biology, genetics, immunology, education, industry, and healthcare fields. The members are committed to research and treatment of endocrine disorders, including diabetes, infertility, osteoporosis, thyroid disease, and obesity and lipid abnormalities.

The Society has developed Clinical Practice Guidelines that are offered to clinicians as the most recent advances and new strategies to improve care by reducing variations in practice, reducing medical errors, and providing consistent quality of care for diagnosing and treating obese or overweight patients. The Society selects topics for guidelines by examining areas where there are no guidelines or where existing guidelines are out of date. Each guideline is created by a task force of experts who rely on evidence-based reviews of the literature to provide support for the recommendations. The Society Web site supplies information about obesity surgery, including the conditions that affect long-term success.

International Food Information Council

The International Food Information Council (IFIC) provides information on food safety, nutrition, and health to health professionals, educators, journalists, and government officials who are responsible for relaying this information to the public. They examine the latest research and break it down into understandable information for the general public. The IFIC media guide on food safety and nutrition lists experts and their contacts with a number of different specialties.

IFIC is supported by the food, beverage, and agricultural industries. They produce a bimonthly newsletter on current topics in food safety and nutrition. The IFIC Web site has resources that are understandable and useful for consumers and health professionals. There is a glossary of food related terms, brochures and fact sheets, videos on current health topics, and a newsroom filled with the latest health information. IFIC developed a partnership with America on the Move, the Food Marketing Institute, and the Presidents Council on Physical Fitness and Sports to create Kidnetics. This is a Web site program for kids and their parents to learn about nutrition and health in a fun and interactive way. It provides kid friendly recipes, games, and physical activity ideas.

IFIC is based in Washington, D.C., and focuses primarily on U.S. issues; however, it also contributes to an informal network of food information organizations in Europe, Asia, Australia, Canada, Japan, New Zealand, and South Africa.

Institute of Medicine of the National Academies of Science

The National Academy of Sciences, signed into being by President Abraham Lincoln (1863), was mandated to "investigate, examine, experiment, and report upon any subject of science or art whenever called upon to do so by any department of the government." NAS eventually expanded to include the National Research Council (1916), National Academy of Engineering (1964), and the Institute of Medicine (IOM; 1970). Collectively, the organizations are known as the National Academies. IOM is a nonprofit organization whose present-day goal is to provide unbiased, science-based information concerning health policy to policy makers, professionals, and the public at large. It publishes reference values for nutrient intakes, such as calories, carbohydrates, and fats, which are periodically updated.

The IOM Web site includes published reports about obesity, including such fact sheets as what the government, industry, and foundations can do to respond to childhood obesity. This page features links to current projects, many of which are devoted to the study of obesity in adults and children.

National Association to Advance Fat Acceptance

National Association to Advance Fat Acceptance (NAAFA) works to eradicate stigma and discrimination based on body size. The tools used are public education, advocacy, and support for association members. It is a forum where issues affecting fat people can be discussed in an unbiased setting. NAAFA provides a legal aid program called FLARE (**F**at **L**egal **A**dvocacy, **R**ights, and **E**ducation) to help people facing size-related discrimination. NAAFA offers members activities and opportunities to get more information and a chance to help the fight against size discrimination. The NAAFA newsletter has up-to-date listings of research, legal and legislative issues, and schedules for the association's meetings and programs. The Fat Activist Task Force encourages letter-writing campaigns that protest or praise advertising and media targets that portray obese people. Local NAAFA chapters throughout the country are led by volunteers and carry out NAAFA's mission at the local level. Most chapters hold local meetings and sponsor workshops and support groups. A wide range of special interest groups (SIGs) within NAAFA that provide programs for members sharing common concerns include: Big Men's Forum, Couples SIG, Diabetic SIG, Military Issues SIG, and Weight Loss Surgery Survivors SIG. Each year NAAFA holds a national meeting that allows members from around the country to network. These meetings present educational and social activities, such as workshops, rallies, sightseeing trips, swim parties, and fashion shows. Specific resources available on the NAAFA Web site include guidelines for health care providers, facts about hypertension, and myths about weight loss and fat people.

The Obesity Society

Founded in 1982 as the North American Society for the Study of Obesity, The Obesity Society (TOS) is the leading scientific society dedicated to the study of obesity. It supports obesity research, education, and advocacy. The organization publishes research on the causes and treatment of obesity, keeps the medical and scientific community and public informed of new advances, and aims to improve the lives of people with obesity. It publishes the journal, *Obesity*.

TOS is committed to advancing public policy changes that focuses on assessment, prevention, and treatment of obesity. TOS advocacy program objectives include: developing programs designed to prevent obesity; ensuring that all people have access to quality medical care for obesity treatment; and increasing funding for obesity research. In pursuing these objectives, TOS works with the U.S. Congress, the U.S. Surgeon General, and CDC.

Robert Wood Johnson Foundation

The Robert Wood Johnson Foundation (RWJF) is a philanthropic organization devoted to improving health policies and practices. It works with individuals, universities, and organizations to address health problems at their roots. RWJF focuses on improving healthcare to help Americans lead healthier lives. The Foundation acknowledges the obesity epidemic in this country by declaring to help reverse it. Their strategies include: investing in research to prevent obesity, action to bring about results, and advocacy to educate policy makers.

RWJF childhood obesity prevention program offers funding for studies that test ways to improve childhood physical activity and nutrition. The Foundation developed the Sports4Kids program, which enables kids to become more physically active at school through organized recreational activities at recess and after school. RWJF is working on bringing affordable and nutritious foods to urban areas nationwide by working with the Philadelphia Food Trust advocacy organization.

Rudd Center for Food Policy & Obesity

Founded in 2005, the Rudd Center for Food Policy & Obesity (RCFPO) is a nonprofit research and public policy organization. Its global goals are to prevent obesity, improve dietary choices, and transform the way in which overweight or obese persons are viewed by the public. To pursue universal health changes, the Center interacts with the media, industry, and government and grassroots activists. It depends upon experts from around the world who represent varied opinions about obesity-related issues in science, law, business, and bioethics. It describes its work as being at the intersection of science and public policy. The Rudd Center's current research studies are designed to increase understanding of the factors that affect how we eat, how we discriminate against overweight and obese people, and how we can change.

Through its Web site, details of these studies and information about obesity are available to the general public, healthcare professionals, policy makers, schools, and educators. Podcasts, handouts, faculty presentations, and a free monthly newsletter are also some of the resources.

Shape Up America!

Shape Up America! (SUA!) is a national initiative founded in 1994 by former Surgeon General C. Everett Koop to promote awareness of obesity as a major public health priority and to provide responsible information on healthy weight management. Its mission is based on the scientific evidence that obesity is a serious health condition and not just an appearance problem. The organization aims to increase cooperation among national and community organizations to make healthy weight and increased physical activity a possibility for all Americans. It seeks to educate the public on how to achieve a healthful weight through increased physical activity and healthy eating. The SUA! Web site is designed to give information to the public, health care professionals, educators, and the media. The professional center contains tools and reports on obesity assessment, treatment, and monitoring. For individuals, there are interactive assessment tools, meal planning guides, and recipes. The *Parents Guide for the Assessment and Treatment of the Overweight Child* provides helpful information for a parent or caregiver of an overweight child on how to increase the chances of successful weight management. A key message is that treatment of childhood obesity should improve the lifestyle of the entire family and not just focus on the child. Ideas and tips for achieving that goal are included in the *Guide*.

Shaping America's Youth

Shaping America's Youth (SAY) is an innovative public and private effort to identify and centralize information on what is being done across America to reverse the rapidly increasing prevalence of overweight and inactivity among children and adolescents. SAY's goal is to provide the latest and most comprehensive information on community efforts that are directed at improving the health of the nation's youth. SAY holds town hall meetings to talk with parents and children to find out what information they want and need to create a community-based action plan.

SAY was developed and is managed by Academic Network. Its Web site has an online survey to collect demographic and funding information about programs throughout the United States that strive to improve childhood nutrition and physical activity. SAY is a National Clearinghouse for this collected information. The site also offers the childhood obesity funding opportunities, publications, schedules of SAY Town Meetings, and other resources related to childhood obesity.

Trust for America's Health

Trust for America's Health (TFAH) is a nonprofit, nonpartisan organization that works to make disease prevention a national priority. It supports a strong and responsive public health system that is vital for preventing disease. On the Web site, the yearly Public Policy Priorities are set forth. Each year, TFAH produces a report on the national status of obesity entitled *The State of Obesity*, which includes a review of federal and state obesity policies and obesity facts for each state. The *State of Your Health* for individual states include: obesity rates in adults and children, hypertension rates, diabetes rates, and percentages of adults who are physically inactive and well as per capita medical costs of obesity.

Veterans Administration National Center for Health Promotion and Disease Prevention

This program seeks to improve the health of veterans and their families across the country. A particular focus is placed on obesity and diabetes, since they are major health concerns for veterans and the VA health care system. The My HealtheVet link offers tools for tracking food intake and physical activity. The Toolkit on the Web site provides a guide for local and state-based VA agencies to implement programs such as The

MOVE! Weight Management Program. It is a patient-centered plan that is intended to help veterans lose weight and keep it off. Other features on the Web site are brochures and video segments. There is also an online library.

World Obesity

World Obesity is an international organization that serves as an umbrella for 52 national obesity associations representing 56 countries. It works for development of effective policies for obesity prevention and management throughout the world. There is an obesity experts forum on the site as well as links to journals specializing in research on obesity and related health problems. It publishes the *International Journal of Obesity*, the *International Journal of Pediatric Obesity*, and *Obesity Reviews*. Another of the Web site features is "Latest News" that provides links to relevant activities and meeting of organizations that are doing obesity research.

Servings Per Co...
Children Under...

Amount Per Serving	Cheerios
	100
Calories	15
Calories from Fat	
	% Da...
	3%
	3%
Total Fat 2g*	
Saturated Fat 0.5g	
Trans Fat 0g	
Polyunsaturated Fat 0.5g	
Monounsaturated Fat 0.5g	0%
Cholesterol 0mg	6%
Sodium 140mg	5%
Potassium 180mg	7%
Total Carbohydrate 20g	11%
Dietary Fiber 3g	
Soluble Fiber 1g	
Sugars 1g	
Other Carbohydrate 16g	
Protein 3g	

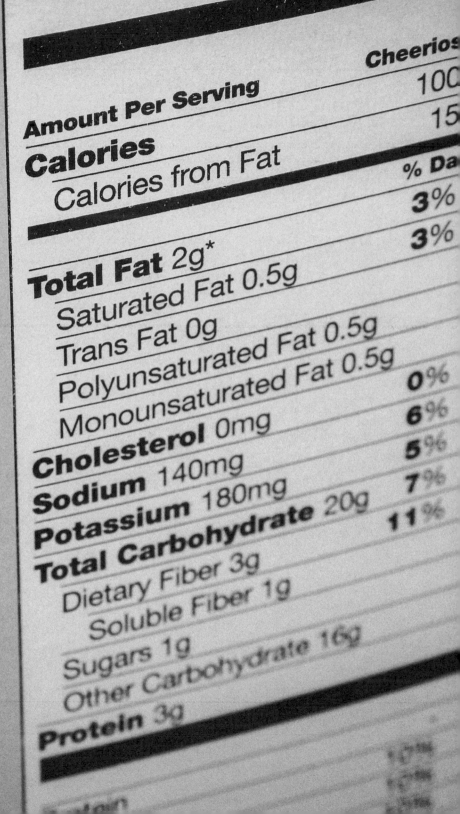

This chapter provides surprising facts related to obesity, as well as graphic figures and tables that depict some of the points made in previous chapters. Also included are excerpts of key documents from the Office of the Surgeon General, Centers for Disease Control and Prevention, and the National Institutes of Health. These documents influence how we view, prevent, and treat obesity.

An extension of research recommendations, federal guidelines, and calls to action new policies, including laws, regulations, and standards, have been designed to encourage a change in the dietary habits of Americans. We include examples of laws that have attempted to define which foods are healthful and which professionals should be endorsed as reliable nutrition experts.

Data

Listed here are selected facts about obesity that were current as of 2014. More detailed information about each of these items is in Chapters 1 and 2.

- It is estimated that more than two-thirds (69%) of adult Americans are overweight and 35 percent are obese (Ogden 2014).

- Childhood obesity has more than doubled in children and quadrupled in adolescents since 1980 (CDC 2014).

Providing nutrition information about foods is an established means of guiding consumers toward more healthful food choices. Federal guidelines, such as the Nutrition Facts Label, have been designed to encourage a change in the dietary habits of Americans. (AP Photo/J. David Ake)

- Non-Hispanic blacks have the highest age-adjusted rates of obesity (47.8%), followed by Hispanics (42.5%), non-Hispanic whites (32.6%), and non-Hispanic Asians (10.8%) (Ogden 2014).

- Obesity is higher among middle age adults, 40–59 years old (39.5%), than among younger adults, age 20–39 (30.3%), or adults 60 or above (35.4%) (Ogden 2014).

- In 2000, a historical moment occurred when the estimated number of overweight people in the world exceeded the number of people suffering from malnutrition (Gardner 2000).

- At least 42 million children under the age of 5 were overweight or obese in 2013, up from 20 million in 2008 (WHO 2015).

- Overweight and obesity increases risk for developing over 35 major diseases, heart disease, hypertension, type 2 diabetes, respiratory problems, osteoarthritis, gallbladder disease, as well as certain types of cancer (NHLBI 1998).

- New technologies at home and on the job and increased sedentary activities, especially television viewing, have reduced the American's need and opportunities to be active. Physical activity levels in the United States have dropped by as much as 32 percent in just two generations (Ng 2012).

- One pound of body fat stores about 3,500 calories.

- A 15-minute brisk walk uses about 100 calories of energy.

- A Burger King Double Whopper with Cheese contains about 1,000 calories ("Burger King U.S. Nutritional Information Core Menu Items January 2014").

- A 24-ounce Jack in the Box Strawberry Shake with Whipped Topping provides almost 1,100 calories (Jack in the Box *Nutritional Facts* 2014).

- In the 1950s, the standard size Coca Cola was about 6 ounces. At many U.S. convenience stores, a 64-ounce soft drinks (2 quarts) are common.

- The success rate for dieting is approximately 3–5 percent (NHLBI 1998).

- At this time, there is no reliable data to show that any diet plan will work better than the others over the long term (Johnston 2014).

- An NIH report shows that bariatric surgical procedures result in greater weight loss than nonsurgical treatments in obese patients over the long term (Courcoulas 2014).

- A randomized, controlled trial reported that skipping breakfast leads to more (not less) weight loss (Levitsky 2013).

- In a laboratory experiment, participants using a small plate did not decrease energy intake but did decrease vegetable intake. Reducing plate size may not promote weight loss. Rather, using a large plate might be a simple strategy to increase vegetable consumption (Libotte 2014).

- Certain intestinal bacteria may cause or protect against obesity. Composition of gut microbes has been shown to differ in lean and obese humans and to change rapidly in response to dietary factors (Tagliabue 2013).

- Insufficient sleep may contribute to overweight and obesity. Increased food intake is a physiological adaptation to provide the body with the energy to sustain extended wakefulness (Markwald 2013).

- Action-related television shows increase food intake. The more distracting a TV show, the less attention people pay to eating, and the more they eat (Tal 2014).

Sources:

Burger King U.S. Nutritional Information Core Menu Items. Accessed January 10, 2014. http://www.bk.com/pdfs/nutrition.pdf.

CDC. "Childhood Obesity Facts." Accessed December 15, 2014. http://www.cdc.gov/healthyyouth/obesity/facts.htm.

Courcoulas, A. P., S. Z. Yanovski, D. Bonds, T. L. Eggerman, M. Horlick, M. A. Staten, and D. E. Arterburn. "Long-Term Outcomes of Bariatric Surgery: A National Institutes of Health symposium." *The Journal of the*

American Medical Association Surgery 149, no. 12 (2014):1323–1329.

Gardner, G., and B. Halweil. *Overfed and Underfed: The Global Epidemic of Malnutrition.* Edited by Jane A. Peterson. Washington, D.C.: Worldwatch Institute, 2000.

Jack in the Box Nutritional Facts. Accessed January 10, 2014. http://assets.jackinthebox.com/pdf_attachment_settings/106/value/Nutritional_Facts.pdf.

Johnston, B. C., S. Kanters, K. Bandayrel, P. Wu, F. Naji, R. A. Siemieniuk, G. D. Ball, J. W. Busse, K. Thorlund, G. Guyatt, J. P. Jansen, and E. J. Mills. "Comparison of Weight Loss among Named Diet Programs in Overweight and Obese Adults: A Meta-Analysis." *The Journal of the American Medical Association* 312, no. 9 (2014): 923–933.

Levitsky, D. A., and C. R. Pacanowski. "Effect of Skipping Breakfast on Subsequent Energy Intake." *Physiology and Behavior* 119 (July 2013): 9–16.

Libotte, E., M. Siegrist, and T. Bucher. "The Influence of Plate Size on Meal Composition. Literature Review and Experiment." *Appetite* 82 (Nov. 2014): 91–96.

Markwald, R. R., E. L. Melanson, M. R. Smith, J. Higgins, L. Perreault, R. H. Eckel, and K. P. Wright, Jr. "Impact of Insufficient Sleep on Total Daily Energy Expenditure, Food Intake, and Weight Gain." *Proceedings of the National Academy of Sciences of the United States of America* 110, no. 14 (2013): 5695–5700.

National Heart, Lung, and Blood Institute (NHLBI). *Clinical Guidelines on the Identification, Evaluation, and Treatment of Overweight and Obesity in Adults: Executive Summary.* Bethesda, MD: National Institutes of Health, 1998.

Ng, S. W., and B. M. Popkin. "Time Use and Physical Activity: A Shift Away from Movement Across the Globe." *Obesity Reviews* 13, no. 8 (2012): 659–680.

Ogden, C. L., M. D. Carroll, B. K. Kit, and K. M. Flegal. "Prevalence of Childhood and Adult Obesity in the United

States, 2011–2012." *The Journal of the American Medical Association* 311, no. 8 (2014): 806–814.

Tagliabue, A., and M. Elli. "The Role of Gut Microbiota in Human Obesity: Recent Findings and Future Perspectives." *Nutrition, Metabolism, and Cardiovascular Diseases* 23, no. 3 (2013): 160–168.

Tal, A., S. Zuckerman, and B. Wansink. "Watch What You Eat: Action-Related Television Content Increases Food Intake." *The Journal of the American Medical Association Internal Medicine* 174, no. 11 (2014): 1842–1843.

World Health Organization (WHO). "World Health Organization. Obesity and Overweight Fact Sheet No. 311." 2015. Accessed February 20, 2015. http://www.who.int/mediacentre/factsheets/fs311/en/.

From 1960 to 2012, the percentage of overweight individuals in U.S. population has remained fairly stable, while those classified with obesity or extreme obesity has continued to rise (see Figure 5.1). Extreme obesity, being 100 or 200 pounds or more overweight with a BMI of over 40 or 50, is associated with complex health issues when compared with moderately obese individuals (BMI 30–35).

More than 40 percent of U.S. food expenditures go toward eating away from home (see Figure 5.2). Lack of time and knowledge of how to prepare food at home contributes to the trend. Other influences are: women employed outside the home, more affordable and convenient food outlets, and increased promotion of restaurant and on-the-go meals. Federal dietary guidelines, such as the Dietary Guidelines for Americans 2010 and Healthy People 2010, now take into account the amounts and nutritional quality of food prepared away from home to develop recommendations.

The algorithm in Figure 5.3 depicts the NHLBI Expert Panel's treatment decision process that provides a step-by-step approach to managing overweight and obese patients.

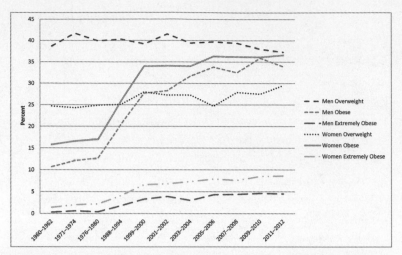

Figure 5.1 Trends in adult overweight, obesity, and extreme obesity among men and women aged 20–74: United States, selected years 1960–1962 through 2011–2012.
Notes: Overweight is body mass index (BMI) greater than or equal to 25.0 kg/m². and less than 30.0 kg/m². Obese is BMI greater than or equal to 30.0 kg/m². Extremely obese is BMI greater than or equal to 40.0 kg/m².
Source: Fryer, C.D. "Prevalence of Overweight, Obesity, and Extreme Obesity among Adults: United States, 1960–1962 through 2011–2012." Centers for Disease Control and Prevention. Accessed December 15, 2014. http://www.cdc.gov/nchs/data/hestat/obesity_adult_11_12/obesity_adult_11_12.htm.

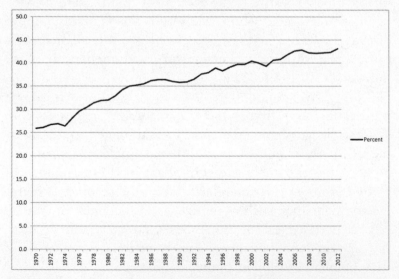

Figure 5.2 Food away-from-home expenditures divided by total food expenditures, for all families and individuals.
Source: Economic Research Service (ERS), U.S. Department of Agriculture (USDA), Food Expenditures. Accessed December 14, 2014. http://www.ers.usda.gov/topics/food-choices-health/food-consumption-demand/food-away-from-home.aspx.

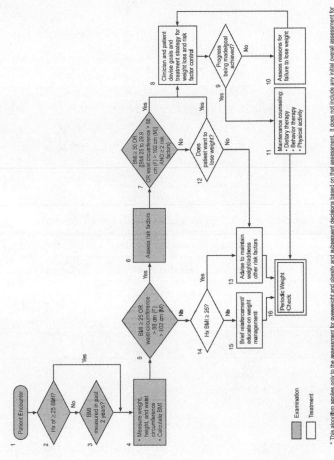

Figure 5.3 Algorithm for the assessment and treatment of overweight and obesity.

Source: NHLBI Obesity Education Initiative Expert Panel on the Identification, Evaluation, and Treatment of Obesity in Adults (United States). *Clinical Guidelines on the Identification, Evaluation, and Treatment of Overweight and Obesity in Adults: The Evidence Report.* Bethesda, MD: National Heart, Lung, and Blood Institute; September 1998. Chapter 4, Treatment Guidelines. Available at: http://www.ncbi.nlm.nih.gov/books/NBK2004/.

The 1942/1943 Metropolitan Life standard height-weight tables for women and men, shown in Tables 5.1 and 5.2, transformed from a record of national averages of weight in relation to age, sex, and height, became widely used for determining "ideal" body weights (MLIC 1942, 1943).

BMI equals a person's weight in kilograms divided by height in meters squared (BMI=kg/m²). Table 5.3 already has the math done. To use the table, find the appropriate height in the left-hand column. Move across the row to the given weight. The number at the top of the column is the BMI for that height and weight. Overweight is defined as a BMI of equal to or greater than 25. Obesity is defined as a BMI of 30 and above. A BMI of 30 is about 30 pounds overweight.

Table 5.1   1943 Metropolitan Life Height and Weight Table for Women

Height (with shoes)	Weight in Pounds (as ordinarily dressed)		
	Small Frame	Medium Frame	Large Frame
5' 0"	105–13	112–20	119–29
5' 1"	107–15	114–22	121–31
5' 2"	110–18	117–25	124–35
5' 3"	113–21	120–23	127–38
5' 4"	116–25	124–32	131–42
5' 5"	119–28	127–35	133–45
5' 6"	123–32	130–40	138–50
5' 7"	126–36	134–44	142–54
5' 8"	129–39	137–47	145–58
5' 9"	133–43	141–51	149–62
5' 10"	136–47	145–55	152–66
5' 11"	139–50	148–58	155–69
6' 0"	141–53	151–63	160–74

Source: MLIC. 1943. Metropolitan Life Insurance Company. Ideal Weights for Women, edited by Metropolitan Life Insurance.

Table 5.2   1942 Metropolitan Life Height and Weight Table for Men

Height (with shoes)	Weight in pounds (as ordinarily dressed)		
	Small Frame	Medium Frame	Large Frame
5' 2"	116–25	124–33	131–42
5' 3"	119–28	127–36	133–44
5' 4"	122–32	130–40	137–49
5' 5"	126–36	134–44	141–53
5' 6"	129–39	137–47	145–57
5' 7"	133–43	141–51	149–62
5' 8"	136–47	145–56	153–66
5' 9"	140–51	149–60	157–70
5' 10"	144–55	153–64	161–75
5' 11"	148–59	157–68	165–80
6' 0"	152–64	161–73	169–85
6' 1"	157–69	166–78	174–90
6' 2"	163–75	171–84	179–96
6' 3"	168–80	176–89	134–202

Source: MLIC. 1942. Metropolitan Insurance Company Ideal Weights for Men, edited by Metropolitan Life Insurance Company.

Skinfold equations estimate body composition from the caliper measurements, which is then used in the Siri equation to estimate percent fat. The Jackson and Pollock (1978) equation for men and Jackson, Pollock, and Ward (1980) for women have been extensively cross-validated with other body composition measures (see Table 5.4). Standard errors range from 3.6 percent to 3.8 percent. The potential errors are increased when these equations are used on populations who are young or old, very lean and muscular, or obese. Body density is estimated by using the skinfold measurements in these equations. In women, the triceps, suprailiac, and thigh skinfolds are measured and in men the chest, abdominal, and thigh skinfolds are used.

Table 5.3 Body Mass Index (BMI) Chart

BMI	19	20	21	22	23	24	25	26	27	28	29	30	31	32	33	34	35
Height (inches)								Body Weight (pounds)									
58	91	96	100	105	110	115	119	124	129	134	138	143	148	153	158	162	167
59	94	99	104	109	114	119	124	128	133	138	143	148	153	158	163	168	173
60	97	102	107	112	118	123	128	133	138	143	148	153	158	163	168	174	179
61	100	106	111	116	122	127	132	137	143	148	153	158	164	169	174	180	185
62	104	109	115	120	126	131	136	142	147	153	158	164	169	175	180	186	191
63	107	113	118	124	130	135	141	146	152	158	163	169	175	180	186	191	197
64	110	116	122	128	134	140	145	151	157	163	169	174	180	186	192	197	204
65	114	120	126	132	138	144	150	156	162	168	174	180	186	192	198	204	210
66	118	124	130	136	142	148	155	161	167	173	179	186	192	198	204	210	216
67	121	127	134	140	146	153	159	166	172	178	185	191	198	204	211	217	223
68	125	131	138	144	151	158	164	171	177	184	190	197	203	210	216	223	230
69	128	135	142	149	155	162	169	176	182	189	196	203	209	216	223	230	236
70	132	139	146	153	160	167	174	181	188	195	202	209	216	222	229	236	243
71	136	143	150	157	165	172	179	186	193	200	208	215	222	229	236	243	250
72	140	147	154	162	169	177	184	191	199	206	213	221	228	235	242	250	258
73	144	151	159	166	174	182	189	197	204	212	219	227	235	242	250	257	265
74	148	155	163	171	179	186	194	202	210	218	225	233	241	249	256	264	272
75	152	160	168	176	184	192	200	208	216	224	232	240	248	256	264	272	279
76	156	164	172	180	189	197	205	213	221	230	238	246	254	263	271	279	287

BMI	36	37	38	39	40	41	42	43	44	45	46	47	48	49	50	51	52	53	54
Height (inches)								Body Weight (pounds)											
58	172	177	181	186	191	196	201	205	210	215	220	224	229	234	239	244	248	253	258
59	178	183	188	193	198	203	208	212	217	222	227	232	237	242	247	252	257	262	267
60	184	189	194	199	204	209	215	220	225	230	235	240	245	250	255	261	266	271	276
61	190	195	201	206	211	217	222	227	232	238	243	248	254	259	264	269	275	280	285
62	196	202	207	213	218	224	229	235	240	246	251	256	262	267	273	278	284	289	295
63	203	208	214	220	225	231	237	242	248	254	259	265	270	278	282	287	293	299	304
64	209	215	221	227	232	238	244	250	256	262	267	273	279	285	291	296	302	308	314
65	216	222	228	234	240	246	252	258	264	270	276	282	288	294	300	306	312	318	324
66	223	229	235	241	247	253	260	266	272	278	284	291	297	303	309	315	322	328	334
67	230	236	242	249	255	261	268	274	280	287	293	299	306	312	319	325	331	338	344
68	236	243	249	256	262	269	276	282	289	295	302	308	315	322	328	335	341	348	354
69	243	250	257	263	270	277	284	291	297	304	311	318	324	331	338	345	351	358	365
70	250	257	264	271	278	285	292	299	306	313	320	327	334	341	348	355	362	369	376
71	257	265	272	279	286	293	301	308	315	322	329	338	343	351	358	365	372	379	386
72	265	272	279	287	294	302	309	316	324	331	338	346	353	361	368	375	383	390	397
73	272	280	288	295	302	310	318	325	333	340	348	355	363	371	378	386	393	401	408
74	280	287	295	303	311	319	326	334	342	350	358	365	373	381	389	396	404	412	420
75	287	295	303	311	319	327	335	343	351	359	367	375	383	391	399	407	415	423	431
76	295	304	312	320	328	336	344	353	361	369	377	385	394	402	410	418	426	435	443

Source: Body Mass Index table. National Heart, Lung, and Blood Institute. Available at: http://www.nhlbi.nih.gov/health/educational/lose_wt/BMI/bmi_tbl.htm.

Table 5.4   Determining Percentage Body Fat Using Skinfold Calipers

Females: Body Density = 1.0994921–0.0009929*sum + 0.0000023*sum^2–
0.0001392*age

(sum means the sum of triceps, suprailiac, thigh skinfold measurements)

Males: Body Density = 1.1093800–0.0008267*sum + 0.0000016*sum^2–
0.0002574*age

(sum means the sum of chest, abdominal, thigh skinfold measurements)

* = times (multiplied by)

How to Measure Body Area Skinfolds

Chest—A diagonal pinch half way between the armpit and the nipple.

Suprailiac—A diagonal pinch just above the front forward protrusion of the hip bone.

Abdominal—A vertical pinch about one inch from your belly button.

Thigh—A vertical pinch halfway between the knee and top of the thigh.

Triceps—A vertical pinch halfway between the shoulder and the elbow.

Estimation of Percent Fat with Siri Equation

(Body density can be determined with skinfold measurements.)

Siri Percent Fat = [(495/Body Density) –450] * 100

A commonly used equation for estimating percent fat from body density is the Siri (1961) formula. A limitation to this formula is that it assumes the density of fat-free mass to remain a constant across the population. Actual percent fat tends to be slightly higher than the measured percent in the lean, muscular individuals and lower in obese individuals.

Sources:

Jackson, A. S., and M. L. Pollock. "Generalized Equations for Predicting Body Density of Men." *British Journal of Nutrition* 40, no. 3 (1078): 497–504.

Jackson, A. S., M. L. Pollock, and A. Ward. "Generalized Equations for Predicting Body Density of Women." *Medicine & Science in Sports & Exercise* 12, no. 3 (1980): 175–181.

Siri, W. E. "Body Composition from Fluid Spaces and Density: Analysis of Methods, 1961." *Nutrition* 9, no. 5 (1993): 480–491; discussion 480, 492.

For estimated amounts of calories needed to maintain calorie balance for various gender and age groups at three different levels of physical activity, see Table 5.5. The estimates are rounded to the nearest 200 calories for assignment to a USDA Food Pattern. An individual's calorie needs may be higher or lower than these average estimates.

Table 5.5 USDA Estimated Calorie Needs per Day by Age, Gender, and Physical Activity Level

| Activity Level | Male | | | Female | | |
	Sedentary	Moderately Active	Active	Sedentary	Moderately Active	Active
Age (years)						
2	1,000	1,000	1,000	1,000	1,000	1,000
3	1,200	1,400	1,400	1,000	1,200	1,400
4	1,200	1,400	1,600	1,200	1,400	1,400
5	1,200	1,400	1,600	1,200	1,400	1,600
6	1,400	1,600	1,800	1,200	1,400	1,600
7	1,400	1,600	1,800	1,200	1,600	1,800
8	1,400	1,600	2,000	1,400	1,600	1,800
9	1,600	1,800	2,000	1,400	1,600	1,800
10	1,600	1,800	2,200	1,400	1,800	2,000
11	1,800	2,000	2,200	1,600	1,800	2,000
12	1,800	2,200	2,400	1,600	2,000	2,200

(Continued)

Table 5.5 (Continued)

Activity Level	Male			Female		
	Sedentary	Moderately Active	Active	Sedentary	Moderately Active	Active
	Age (years)					
13	2,000	2,200	2,600	1,600	2,000	2,200
14	2,000	2,400	2,800	1,800	2,000	2,400
15	2,200	2,600	3,000	1,800	2,000	2,400
16	2,400	2,800	3,200	1,800	2,000	2,400
17	2,400	2,800	3,200	1,800	2,000	2,400
18	2,400	2,800	3,200	1,800	2,000	2,400
19–20	2,600	2,800	3,000	2,000	2,200	2,400
21–25	2,400	2,800	3,000	2,000	2,200	2,400
26–30	2,400	2,600	3,000	1,800	2,000	2,400
31–35	2,400	2,600	3,000	1,800	2,000	2,200
36–40	2,400	2,600	2,800	1,800	2,000	2,200
41–45	2,200	2,600	2,800	1,800	2,000	2,200
46–50	2,200	2,400	2,800	1,800	2,000	2,200
51–55	2,200	2,400	2,800	1,600	1,800	2,200
56–60	2,200	2,400	2,600	1,600	1,800	2,200
61–65	2,000	2,400	2,600	1,600	1,800	2,000
66–70	2,000	2,200	2,600	1,600	1,800	2,000
71–75	2,000	2,200	2,600	1,600	1,800	2,000
76+	2,000	2,200	2,400	1,600	1,800	2,000

a. Based on Estimated Energy Requirements (EER) equations, using reference heights (average) and reference weights (healthy) for each age-gender group. For children and adolescents, reference height and weight vary. For adults, the reference man is 5 feet 10 inches tall and weighs 154 pounds. The reference woman is 5 feet 4 inches tall and weighs 126 pounds. EER equations are from the Institute of Medicine. *Dietary Reference Intakes for Energy, Carbohydrate, Fiber, Fat, Fatty Acids, Cholesterol, Protein, and Amino Acids*. Washington D.C.: The National Academies Press, 2002.

b. Sedentary means a lifestyle that includes only the light physical activity associated with typical day-to-day life. Moderately active means a lifestyle that includes physical activity equivalent to walking about 1.5–3 miles per day at 3–4 miles per hour, in addition to the light physical activity associated with typical day-to-day life. Active means a lifestyle that includes physical activity equivalent to walking more than 3 miles per day at 3–4 miles per hour, in addition to the light physical activity associated with typical day-to-day life.

c. Estimates for females do not include women who are pregnant or breastfeeding.

Source: Center for Nutrition Policy and Promotion. Available at: http://www.cnpp .usda.gov/sites/default/files/usda_food_patterns/EstimatedCalorieNeedsPer DayTable.pdf.

The Food Patterns in Table 5.6 suggest amounts of food to consume from the basic food groups, subgroups, and oils to meet recommended nutrient intakes at 12 different calorie levels. Nutrient and energy contributions from each group are calculated according to the nutrient-dense forms of foods in each group (e.g., lean meats and fat-free milk). The table also shows the number of calories from solid fats and added sugars (SoFAS) that can be accommodated within each calorie level, in addition to the suggested amounts of nutrient-dense forms of foods in each group.

Table 5.7 is an example of how to keep track of foods eaten during the day. Table 5.8 helps sort through the various types of diets that exist today. It lists some of the most common diet plans, examines the advantages and disadvantages, and the dietary basis behind their potential benefits.

Table 5.6 USDA Pyramid Food Intake Patterns, Daily Amount of Food from Each Group

Calorie Level	1,000	1,200	1,400	1,600	1,800	2,000	2,200	2,400	2,600	2,800	3,000	3,200
Fruits	1 cup	1 cup	1 cup	1½ cups	1½ cups	1½ cups	2 cups	2 cups	2 cups	2 cups	2½ cups	2½ cups
Vegetables	1 cup	1½ cups	1½ cups	2 cups	2½ cups	2½ cups	3 cups	3 cups	3½ cups	3½ cups	4 cups	4 cups
Grains	3 oz-eq	4 oz-eq	5 oz-eq	5 oz-eq	6 oz-eq	6 oz-eq	7 oz-eq	8 oz-eq	9 oz-eq	10 oz-eq	10 oz-eq	10 oz-eq
Protein Foods	2 oz-eq	3 oz-eq	4 oz-eq	5 oz-eq	5 oz-eq	5½ oz-eq	6 oz-eq	6½ oz-eq	6½ oz-eq	7 oz-eq	7 oz-eq	7 oz-eq
Dairy	2 cups	2 cups	2½ cups	2½ cups	3 cups	3 cups	3 cups	3 cups	3 cups	3 cups	3 cups	3 cups
Oils	15 g	17 g	17 g	22 g	24 g	27 g	29 g	31 g	34 g	36 g	44 g	51 g
Limit on calories from SoFAS	137	121	121	121	161	258	266	330	362	395	459	596

Source: Center for Nutrition Policy and Promotion. Available at: http://www.cnpp.usda.gov/sites/default/files/usda_food_patterns/USDAFoodPatternsSummaryTable.pdf.

Table 5.7   Daily Food Record Form

Time	Amount	Food Eaten	How Prepared	How Hungry Am I? 0 = not hungry 5 = very hungry
6 am	1 cup	1 percent milk		1
	2 cups	Cheerios		
	2 tablespoons	White sugar		
	2 c	Black coffee	Brewed	
	2 tablespoons	Fat-free non-dairy creamer	In coffee	
10 am	2–3 inch diameter	Chocolate chip cookies	From grocery bakery	3
Noon	2 slices	Ham, deli sliced	In sandwich	4
	1 slice	American cheese	In sandwich	
	1 leaf 2 slices	Iceberg lettuce, 2 pickle slices	In sandwich	
	1 tsp	Mustard	In sandwich	
	2 tablespoons	Kraft real mayo	In sandwich	
	2 slices	Orowheat 100 percent whole wheat bread	In sandwich	
	1 bag (1.4 oz)	Doritos corn chips		
	16 ounces	Sprite	Bottle	
5 pm	2 c	Lasagna noodles with meat Stouffer's frozen dinner	Baked	4
	2 slices	White Italian bread	Toasted	
	2 teaspoons	Promise light margarine	Spread on toast	
8 pm	2 cups	Ben and Jerry's vanilla ice cream	In bowl	2

Table 5.8　Types of Diet Plans with Claims and Advantages

Diet Plan Characteristics	Examples	Claims/Advantages
Calorie controlled, low fat, high carbohydrates	Weight Watchers, Volumetrics, Ornish, Pritikin	Balanced plan Ease into maintenance
High protein, high fat, low carbohydrates	Atkins, Scarsdale, Carb Addicts, Sugar Busters Quick Weight Loss, Protein power, South Beach—initial stage	Quick initial weight loss No measuring No hunger
High protein, moderate fat, moderate carbohydrates	Zone, South Beach—later stages	Use fat for energy No hunger Include a wide variety of foods
Meal replacement	Jenny Craig, Nutrasystems	Portion controlled No meal preparation
Liquid protein shakes/ bars	Optifast, Medifast, Health Maintenance Resources, Cambridge, Slimfast	Minimal dealing with food Quick initial weight loss
Others: May have very specific recommendations that make them unique; however, diet composition is generally similar to low fat or low carbohydrate, low calorie	Fit for Life, Food Combining, Fat flush, Eat for Your Blood Type, Suzanne Sommers	Quick initial weight loss Structured plan

Documents

Government Reports

The Surgeon General's Vision for a Healthy and Fit Nation (2010)

Reports from the United States Surgeon General are intended to heighten the nation's awareness of important public health issues and to generate major public health initiatives. For example, reports on the adverse health consequences of smoking triggered nationwide efforts to prevent tobacco use. A Surgeon General's Call to Action report is a science-based document meant to stimulate action to solve a major public health problem such as obesity.

*In 2001, Surgeon General David Satcher, M.D., Ph.D., is-*sued A Call to Action to Prevent and Decrease Overweight and Obesity *that warned of the negative effects of the increasing weight of Americans and outlined a public health response to reverse the trend. Dr. Satcher declared that the nationwide rise in overweight and obesity was a major public health issue facing the United States. The report emphasized the magnitude of the concern by drawing on statistical data showing the rising trend in obesity and overweight in the United States and used research findings to document the associated health risks and economic impact. Dr. Satcher admitted that "Many people believe that dealing with overweight and obesity is a personal responsibility. To some degree they are right, but it is also a community responsibility."*

Satcher acknowledged that there was no clear evidence on how to effectively prevent and reduce obesity and overweight. He reasoned that this lack of information demanded a concerted national public health response. The Call to Action urged a cooperative effort from individuals, families, communities, schools, work sites, organizations, and the media to set priorities, establish strategies and actions at multiple levels, and provide a starting point for groups and individuals to find new ways to reduce and prevent overweight and obesity.

In 2010, an updated Call released by Surgeon General Regina Benjamin, M.D., M.B.A. was A Vision for a Healthy and Fit Nation. *Dr. Benjamin's message was that, while some headway had been made since the 2001 report, the prevalence of obesity and obesity-related disabilities remained too high. She planned to strengthen and expand the previous blueprint for action and change the focus from a negative one about obesity and health risks to a positive one aimed at being healthy and fit. She proposed that "We need to stop bombarding Americans with what they can't do and what they can't eat. We need to begin to talk about what they can do to become healthy and fit."*

Excerpts from The Surgeon General's Vision for a Healthy and Fit Nation *are included here. The first is her directive to change the focus of obesity treatment to one focusing on positive aspects of nutrition and fitness and a call to all Americans to join the effort. The second includes portions from the Opportunities for Prevention section outlining obesity prevention interventions that focus not only on personal behaviors and biological traits, but also on the social and physical environments that encourage or limit opportunities for positive health outcomes.*

To stop the obesity epidemic in this country, we must remember that Americans will be more likely to change their behavior if they have a meaningful reward—something more than just reaching a certain weight or BMI measurement. The real reward has to be something that people can feel and enjoy and celebrate. That reward is invigorating, energizing, joyous health. It is a level of health that allows people to embrace each day and live their lives to the fullest—without disease, disability, or lost productivity.

Good nutrition, regular physical activity, and stress management significantly contribute to achieving optimal health. By practicing these healthy lifestyle behaviors, excess weight is prevented, weight loss is sustained, and strength and endurance are achieved. This is the reward we need to communicate to the American public. We must help our communities make the important and life-saving connection between being healthy, fit and living well.

We are indeed at a crossroads. The "old normal" was to stress the importance of attaining recommended numbers for weight and BMI. Although these numbers are important measures of disease and disability, the total picture is much bigger. It involves the creation of a "new normal"—an emphasis on achieving an optimal level of health and well-being. People want to live long and live well, and they are making their voices heard across this nation. Today's obesity epidemic calls for committed, compassionate citizens to mobilize and demand the health and well-being they so richly deserve. I have heard this call to arms, and I am honored to do everything in my power to help Americans live long and live well.

. . .

I am calling on all Americans to join me in a national grassroots effort to reverse this trend. My plan includes showing people how to choose nutritious food, add more physical activity to their daily lives, and manage the stress that so often derails their best efforts at developing healthy habits. I envision men, women, and children who are mentally and physically fit to live their lives to the fullest. The real goal is not just a number on a scale, but optimal health for all Americans at every stage of life. To achieve this goal, we must all work together to share resources, educate our citizens, and partner with business and government leaders to find creative solutions in our neighborhoods, towns, and cities from coast to coast. Together, we can become a nation committed to become healthy and fit.

. . .

Opportunities for Prevention

Messages and suggestions for action in the Surgeon General's report A Vision for a Healthy and Fit Nation *are based on research and practice discoveries that have identified the most effective and achievable approaches for improving the health and well-being of Americans. The* Opportunities for Prevention *portion provides knowledge, tools, and options for interventions that can occur in multiple settings as outlined by the section headings:*

> *Individual Healthy Choices and Healthy Home Environments*
> *Creating a Healthy Home Environment*
> *Creating Healthy Child Care Settings*
> *Creating Healthy Schools*
> *Creating Healthy Work Sites*
> *Mobilizing the Medical Community*
> *Improving Our Communities*

The following excerpt includes recommendations that support healthy homes, child care settings, and schools. Descriptions of healthful choices for work sites, medical mobilization, and community improvement can be read in the full report.

Individual Healthy Choices and Healthy Home Environments

As a society, we have to begin to change our habits one healthy choice at a time. Change starts with the individual choices we as Americans make each day for ourselves and those around us. Balancing good nutrition and physical activity while managing daily stressors is always a challenge, but one that can be achieved. Finding time to shop for and prepare healthy meals after work and between family activities requires planning. Stress and a lack of available healthy and affordable foods are some of the reasons why many people turn to fast food as a regular source for meals. Eating excess calories contributes to obesity, but so does watching too much television and sitting for hours in front of a computer.

This fact is especially true for children and teenagers. Technological advancements have made our lives more convenient—but also more sedentary. Research shows that leading an inactive life not only increases the risk of becoming overweight or obese, but also contributes to an increased risk for disease and disability.

The good news is that we can overcome these challenges—and the reward is the creation of a healthy and fit nation. Healthy choices include:

- Reducing consumption of sodas and juices with added sugars.
- Reducing consumption of energy dense foods that primarily contain added sugars or solid fats.
- Eating more fruits, vegetables, whole grains, and lean proteins.
- Controlling your portions.
- Drinking more water.
- Choosing low-fat or non-fat dairy products.
- Limiting television viewing time and consider keeping televisions out of children's rooms.
- Becoming more physically active throughout the day.
- Breastfeeding exclusively to 6 months.

Creating a Healthy Home Environment

As adults, we need to help our children get off to a good start. The earliest risks for childhood obesity begin during pregnancy. Excess weight gain, diabetes, and smoking during pregnancy are not just health risks for the mother—they also put children at risk for obesity early in life. Keeping pregnancy weight gain within recommended limits will help prevent diabetes in the mother. Stopping cigarette smoking and abstaining from alcohol and drug use will protect the health of the mother and the baby.

The earliest decisions regarding food, activity, and television viewing occur in the home. Parents and other caregivers play a key role in making good choices for themselves and their loved one. Children and teenagers look to their mothers and fathers and other caregivers to model healthy lifestyle habits, and adults need to teach by example. In some households, several generations may live together or have responsibility for children at different times during the day. This sharing of duties requires coordination and consistency in activities and habits related to food shopping and preparation, access to physical activity, and limits on television and computer use.

Both young children and teenagers learn from the choices they see adults make. One way to help children learn is to involve all family members in family-based physical activities and in planning, shopping for, and preparing meals. These activities provide both an education in healthy nutrition and exercise, as well as a critical foundation for how to make healthy lifestyle choices.

Healthy Food Choices

The first decision that parents make about what to feed their child occurs during pregnancy. After the baby is born, mothers should breastfeed whenever possible because it provides the highest quality of nutrition and helps to prevent early childhood obesity. By age 2, children should be drinking low-fat or non-fat milk. As parents, we are in charge of the foods we provide to our children. Creativity with food preparation can often solve the problems presented by picky eaters. Adults also should offer children small portions and show them how to eat slowly and enjoy their meal.

Healthy Teenagers

The teenage years present unique challenges. Adolescence is a time of vulnerability to the development of psychiatric disorders, including eating disorders, depression, drug and alcohol abuse. Adolescent boys and girls are subjected to significant peer pressure related to eating and exercise, and most school systems provide limited opportunities for physical activity. Teenagers often drink more carbonated and caffeinated beverages and eat more fast foods. These multiple stresses and unhealthy habits make teenagers particularly vulnerable to becoming sedentary, overweight, and obese. An obese teenager has a greater than 70% risk of becoming an obese adult. Parents should guide their teenagers to become fit and healthy adults while being cautious not to trigger unhealthy eating behaviors or eating disorders.

Physical Activity

Scheduling time for the recommended levels of physical activity is essential to overall health. Physical activity can help control weight, reduce risk for many diseases (heart disease and some cancers), strengthen your bones and muscles, improve your mental health, and increase your chances of living longer.

Adults should do at least 150 minutes of moderate-intensity physical activity per week. Aerobic activity such as brisk walking or general gardening should be done in episodes of at least 10 minutes and preferably should be spread throughout the week. For children and teenagers, the recommendation is for 1 hour of daily physical activity that includes vigorous activities and activities that strengthen their bones.

Making physical activities fun can affect how children and teenagers respond to changes in their routine. Programmed, repetitious exercise may work for adults, but it rarely works for children. Look for ways to add physical activity throughout the day. When possible, parents should walk with children to and from school, and children should have scheduled time to play. Because safety is a real concern in many neighborhoods, citizens should talk with their local elected officials and members of law enforcement to find ways to improve safety so everyone can walk or play outdoors.

Television and Computer Use

In recent years, we have witnessed an explosion of technological advances in televisions, home entertainment centers, computers, and video game players. A new report released in 2010 found that nearly two-thirds of kids aged 8–18 say the TV is usually on during meals and nearly half report the TV is left on "most of the time" in their home. Seven in ten young people have a TV in their bedroom and 50% also have a console video game player in their room. Overall, 8–18 year-olds spend over 7 hours per day using entertainment media (TV, video games, computers) amounting to more than 53 hours a week.

The hours that adults, teenagers, and children are spending in front of a television or computer screen contribute to their sedentary lifestyle and increase their risk for obesity. In particular, the more time children spend watching television, the more likely they are to eat while doing so and the more likely they are to eat the high-calorie food that are heavily advertised to both adults and children.

Most parents either do not set limitations on screen time or don't enforce them. Studies have shown that when parents establish rules and implement them, screen time declines by 2 hours per day, leaving opportunities for more physical activity. Parents need to be role models by limiting their own television time and spending more time with their children.

Creating Healthy Child Care Settings

Early childhood settings, including child care and early childhood education programs, affect the lives of millions of U.S. children. In 2005, 61% of children aged 0–6 years who were not yet in kindergarten (about 12 million children) received some form of child care on a regular basis from someone other than their parents. Child care programs should identify and implement approaches that reflect expert recommendations on physical activity, screen time limitations, good nutrition, and healthy sleep practices. Early childhood providers, like parents, should model healthy lifestyle behaviors and teach children how to make healthy choices. They also should reach out to parents to encourage them to practice and promote healthy habits at home.

To choose a healthy child care environment, parents should:

- Ask childcare providers about their approach to promoting healthy lifestyles for children.
- Visit the setting to see how childcare providers model and teach physical activity, good nutrition, and healthy sleep practices.
- Ask childcare providers how they keep parents informed about what they can do at home to support their child's physical activity, good nutrition, and healthy sleep practices.
- Ask childcare providers about their support of breastfeeding, breast milk storage and handling.

Child care providers should:

- Identify and use resources that recommend effective approaches to promoting physical activity, good nutrition, and healthy sleep in early childhood settings.
- Establish and post policies, procedures, and practices that support these approaches in ways that respect local communities and cultures.
- Stay current in these approaches through required regular training.
- Educate and involve parents in trainings and other activities.

State regulations regarding physical activity, nutrition, and screen time vary greatly among child care settings by state and type (e.g., Head Start, center-based child care, family-based child care). Standardized national goals for early child care—especially ones related to healthy weight—would improve the quality of early childhood settings and give childcare providers and parents a foundation to improve their knowledge and skills to support these goals.

For example, recommended policies that can help child care programs support healthy weight for young children include the following:

- Require 60 minutes of a mix of structured and unstructured daily physical activity.

- Establish nutrition requirements in child care by using national recommendations such as the Dietary Guidelines for Americans.

- Use a structured approach to training child care providers how to promote physical activity and good nutrition and how to educate and involve parents in these activities

- Give parents materials that reinforce the practices of child care settings that promote physical activity and good nutrition and limit screen time.

Creating Healthy Schools

Schools play a pivotal role in preventing obesity among children and teenagers. Each school day provides multiple opportunities for students to learn about health and practice healthy behaviors that affect weight, including physical activity and good nutrition. Well-designed school programs can promote physical activity and healthy eating, reduce the rate of overweight and obesity among children and teenagers, and improve academic achievement.

To ensure that nutrition and physical activity programs are effective, school administrations need physical education specialists, health education specialists, and certified food service staff. Schools should encourage and reinforce healthy dietary behaviors by providing nutritious and appealing foods and beverages in all venues accessible to students, including the cafeteria, vending machines, school stores, and concession stands. A substantial percentage of students' recommended physical activity can be provided through a comprehensive school-based physical activity program that includes high-quality physical education, recess and other physical activity breaks, intramurals and physical activity clubs, interscholastic sports, and walk- and bike-to-school initiatives.

High-quality physical education gives young people a chance to learn the skills needed to establish and maintain physically active lifestyles throughout their lives. States and local school districts set requirements for physical activity levels.

In 2006, few schools provided daily physical education or its equivalent for the entire school year to all students. Nationwide, only 30% of high school students attended physical education classes 5 days in an average school week, compared with 42% in 1991.

To help students develop healthy habits, schools should have comprehensive wellness plans that include:

- An active school health council to guide health-related policy decisions.

- A planned and sequential health education curriculum for pre-kindergarten through grade 12. This curriculum should be based on national standards and address a clear set of behavioral outcomes that empower students to make healthy dietary choices and meet physical activity recommendations.

- A school and school workplace wellness policy that includes teachers and other school employees to model healthy behaviors.

- A comprehensive professional development and credentialing program for staff that addresses health education, physical education, food service, and health services.

- Partnerships with parent-teacher organizations, families, and community members to support healthy eating and physical activity policies and programs.

To promote healthy nutrition, schools should:

- Establish nutrition standards that promote healthy nutritious foods.

- Ensure availability of appealing, healthy food options that enable students to comply with recommendations in the

U.S. Dietary Guidelines for Americans, including fresh fruits and vegetables, whole grains, and lean proteins.

- Use presentation, marketing, and education techniques to encourage students to eat more fruits and vegetables, whole grains, and lean proteins and to drink more water and low-fat or non-fat beverages.
- Make sure water is available throughout the school setting
- Limit amounts of high calorie snack options, including beverages in vending machines.

To promote physical activity, school systems should:

- Require daily physical education for students in pre-kindergarten through grade 12, allowing 150 minutes per week for elementary schools and 225 minutes per week for secondary schools.
- Require and implement a planned and sequential physical education curriculum for pre-kindergarten through grade 12 that is based on national standards.
- Require at least 20 minutes daily recess for all students in elementary schools.
- Offer students opportunities to participate in intramural physical activity programs during after-school hours.
- Implement and promote walk- and bike-to-school programs.
- Establish joint use agreements with local government agencies to allow use of school facilities for physical activity programs offered by the school or community-based organizations outside of school hours.

Source: U.S. Department of Health and Human Services. *The Surgeon General's Vision for a Healthy and Fit Nation*. Rockville, MD: U.S. Department of Health and Human Services, Office of the Surgeon General, 2010. Available at: http://www.surgeongeneral.gov/priorities/healthy-fit-nation/obesityvision2010.pdf.

School Health Guidelines to Promote Healthy Eating and Physical Activity (2011)

Data and reports from the National Center for Health Statistics, the nation's principal health statistics agency that provides data to identify and address health issues, indicate that the percentage of children aged 6–11 years in the United States who were obese increased from 7 percent in 1980 to nearly 18 percent in 2012. The percentage of adolescents aged 12–19 years who were obese increased from 5 percent to nearly 21 percent over the same period. These numbers show that obesity has more than doubled in children and quadrupled in adolescents in the past 30 years.

Children and adolescents who are obese are at greater risk for cardiovascular disease and diabetes, bone and joint difficulties, and social and psychological problems such as stigmatization and poor self-esteem. While positive lifestyle habits, including healthy eating and consistent physical activity, can lower the risk of becoming obese and developing related diseases, behaviors of children and adolescents are influenced by many sectors of society, including families, medical care providers, the media and entertainment industries, food and beverage industries, and schools. Since children and adolescents spend a large part of their day in schools, the setting is one that is well-positioned to help prevent obesity. Through policies, practices, and a supportive environment, schools can provide opportunities for students to learn about and apply healthy eating and physical activity behaviors.

In response to the childhood obesity epidemic, extensive research has been conducted on school-based healthy eating and physical activity promotion. In 2011, the U.S. Centers for Disease Control (CDC) released School Health Guidelines to Promote Healthy Eating and Physical Activity, a report synthesized from up-to-date scientific evidence and best practices by education professionals. The guidelines incorporate the 2010 Dietary Guidelines for Americans, the 2008 Physical Activity Guidelines for Americans, and the Healthy People 2020. The purpose of the report is to provide science-based guidance for schools on establishing a school environment supportive of healthy eating and physical activity.

Nine guidelines are accompanied by specific strategies for schools to implement.

The intended audience for this report is broad. State and local education and health agencies, federal agencies, and national non-governmental organizations, physical education and health education teachers, school nutrition directors, parents, students, and anyone who is interested in the health of students in school. In addition, faculty members in institutions of higher education can use these guidelines to teach students who study public health, physical education, dietetics, nursing, elementary and secondary education, and other health- and education-related disciplines.

To help inform education and health professionals, the CDC developed numerous free training tools to introduce the guidelines to staff members at education and health agencies, schools, community groups, and the general public. A particularly useful module in the guidelines is the practical and readily applicable Tips for Teachers.

The documents included below are examples from the Executive Summary of the Guidelines that provides an overview of the nine guidelines and strategies to accomplish them, and the entire Tips for Teachers module.

Executive Summary

Healthy eating and regular physical activity play a powerful role in preventing chronic diseases, including heart disease, cancer, and stroke—the three leading causes of death among adults aged 18 years or older. Engaging students in healthy eating and regular physical activity can help lower their risk for obesity and related chronic diseases during adulthood.

Schools play a critical role in improving the dietary and physical activity behaviors of students. Schools can create an environment supportive of students' efforts to eat healthily and be active by implementing policies and practices that support healthy eating and regular physical activity and by providing opportunities for students to learn about and practice these behaviors. CDC synthesized research and best practices related to promoting healthy eating and physical activity in schools, culminating in nine guidelines. These guidelines were informed by the Dietary Guidelines for Americans, the Physical Activity Guidelines for Americans,8 and the Healthy People 2020 objectives related to healthy eating and physical activity among children and adolescents, including associated school objectives.

The guidelines serve as the foundation for developing, implementing, and evaluating school-based healthy eating and physical activity policies and practices for students. Each of the nine guidelines is accompanied by a set of implementation strategies developed to help schools work toward achieving each guideline. Although the ultimate goal is to implement all nine guidelines included in this document, not every strategy will be appropriate for every school, and some schools, due to resource limitations, might need to implement the guidelines incrementally.

Guideline 1: Use a coordinated approach to develop, implement, and evaluate healthy eating and physical activity policies and practices.

Representatives from different segments of the school and community, including parents and students, should work together to maximize healthy eating and physical activity opportunities for students.

Strategies
- Coordinate healthy eating and physical activity policies and practices through a school health council and school health coordinator.
- Assess healthy eating and physical activity policies and practices.
- Use a systematic approach to develop, implement, and monitor healthy eating and physical activity policies.
- Evaluate healthy eating and physical activity policies and practices.

Guideline 2: Establish school environments that support healthy eating and physical activity.

The school environment should encourage all students to make healthy eating choices and be physically active throughout the school day.

Strategies

- Provide access to healthy foods and physical activity opportunities and to safe spaces, facilities, and equipment for healthy eating and physical activity.
- Establish a climate that encourages and does not stigmatize healthy eating and physical activity.
- Create a school environment that encourages a healthy body image, shape, and size among all students and staff members, is accepting of diverse abilities, and does not tolerate weight-based teasing.

Guideline 3: Provide a quality school meal program and ensure that students have only appealing, healthy food and beverage choices offered outside of the school meal program.

Schools should model and reinforce healthy dietary behaviors by ensuring that only nutritious and appealing foods and beverages are provided in all food venues in schools, including school meal programs; à la carte service in the cafeteria; vending machines; school stores and snack bars/concession stands; fundraisers on school grounds; classroom-based activities; staff and parent meetings; and after-school programs.

Strategies

- Promote access to and participation in school meals.
- Provide nutritious and appealing school meals that comply with the Dietary Guidelines for Americans.
- Ensure that all foods and beverages sold or served outside of school meal programs are nutritious and appealing.

Guideline 4: Implement a comprehensive physical activity program with quality physical education as the cornerstone.

Children and adolescents should participate in 60 minutes or more of physical activity every day. A substantial percentage of students' physical activity can be provided through a comprehensive, school-based physical activity program that includes these components: physical education, recess, classroom-based physical activity, walking and bicycling to school, and out-of-school-time activities.

Strategies

- Require students in grades K–12 to participate in daily physical education that uses a planned and sequential curriculum and instructional practices that are consistent with national or state standards for physical education.

- Provide a substantial percentage of each student's recommended daily amount of physical activity in physical education class.

- Use instructional strategies in physical education that enhance students' behavioral skills, confidence in their abilities, and desire to adopt and maintain a physically active lifestyle.

- Provide ample opportunities for all students to engage in physical activity outside of physical education class.

- Ensure that physical education and other physical activity programs meet the needs and interests of all students.

Guideline 5: Implement health education that provides students with the knowledge, attitudes, skills, and experiences needed for healthy eating and physical activity.

Health education is integral to the primary mission of schools, providing students with the knowledge and skills they need to become successful learners and healthy adults.

Strategies

- Require health education from pre-kindergarten through grade 12.

- Implement a planned and sequential health education curriculum that is culturally and developmentally appropriate, addresses a clear set of behavioral outcomes that promote healthy eating and physical activity, and is based on national standards.

- Use curricula that are consistent with scientific evidence of effectiveness in helping students improve healthy eating and physical activity behaviors.

- Use classroom instructional methods and strategies that are interactive, engage all students, and are relevant to their daily lives and experiences.

Guideline 6: Provide students with health, mental health, and social services to address healthy eating, physical activity, and related chronic disease prevention.

Schools are responsible for students' physical health, mental health, and safety during the school day. Schools should ensure resources are available for identification, follow-up, and treatment of health and mental health conditions related to diet, physical activity, and weight status.

Strategies

- Assess student needs related to physical activity, nutrition, and obesity, and provide counseling and other services to meet those needs.

- Ensure students have access to needed health, mental health, and social services.

- Provide leadership in advocacy and coordination of effective school physical activity and nutrition policies and practices.

Guideline 7: Partner with families and community members in the development and implementation of healthy eating and physical activity policies, practices, and programs.

Partnerships among schools, families, and community members can enhance student learning, promote consistent messaging about health behaviors, increase resources, and engage, guide, and motivate students to eat healthily and be active.

Strategies

- Encourage communication among schools, families, and community members to promote adoption of healthy eating and physical activity behaviors among students.
- Involve families and community members on the school health council.
- Develop and implement strategies for motivating families to participate in school-based programs and activities that promote healthy eating and physical activity.
- Access community resources to help provide healthy eating and physical activity opportunities for students.
- Demonstrate cultural awareness in healthy eating and physical activity practices throughout the school.

Guideline 8: Provide a school employee wellness program that includes healthy eating and physical activity services for all school staff members.

School employee wellness programs can improve staff productivity, decrease employee absenteeism, and decrease employee health care costs.

Strategies

- Gather data and information to determine the nutrition and physical activity needs of school staff members and assess the availability of existing school employee wellness activities and resources.

- Encourage administrative support for and staff involvement in school employee wellness.

- Develop, implement, and evaluate healthy eating and physical activity programs for all school employees.

Guideline 9: Employ qualified persons, and provide professional development opportunities for physical education, health education, nutrition services, and health, mental health, and social services staff members, as well as staff members who supervise recess, cafeteria time, and out-of-school-time programs.

Providing certified and qualified staff with regular professional development opportunities enables them to improve current skills and acquire new ones.

Strategies

- Require the hiring of physical education teachers, health education teachers, and nutrition services staff members who are certified and appropriately prepared to deliver quality instruction, programs, and practices.

- Provide school staff with annual professional development opportunities to deliver quality physical education, health education, and nutrition services.

- Provide annual professional development opportunities for school health, mental health, and social services staff members, and staff members who lead or supervise out-of-school-time programs, recess, and cafeteria time.

Source: Centers for Disease Control and Prevention. "School Health Guidelines to Promote Healthy Eating and Physical Activity." *Morbidity and Mortality Weekly Report* 60, no. 5, September 16, 2011. Available at: http://www.cdc.gov/healthy youth/npao/strategies.htm.

Tips for Teachers

Allow Access to Drinking Water

Access to drinking water throughout the day gives students a healthy alternative to sugar-sweetened beverages.

Staying hydrated may also improve student cognitive function.

- Allow students to visit the water fountain throughout the school day and to carry water bottles in class.
- Send a note to parents that students will be allowed to bring water bottles to your class, though not mandatory. If bottles are filled at home, ask parents to use only plain water.
- Inform school maintenance staff if water fountains are not clean or are not functioning properly.

Use Student Rewards That Support Health

Children are at risk of associating food with emotions and feelings of accomplishment when food is used in the classroom as a reward. This reinforces the practice of eating outside of meal or snack times and encourages students to eat treats even when they are not hungry. This practice may create lifetime habits of rewarding or comforting oneself with unhealthy eating.

- Do not use food or beverages to reward student achievement or good behavior.
- Avoid giving students candy or food coupons.
- Use nonfood items, activities and opportunities for physical activity to recognize students for their achievements or good behavior.
- Offer stickers, books, extra time for recess, or walks with the principal or teacher.
- Do not withhold food, beverages, or physical activity time to discipline for academic performance or poor classroom behavior.

Make Celebrations and Fundraisers Healthier

- Encourage parents to provide healthy foods and beverages for birthday and classroom parties if food is served.
- Send a note to parents suggesting healthier options, such as fruits, vegetables, or whole grain snacks.
- Consider nonfood celebrations such as guest speakers, an extra recess period, or class games.
- Use healthy foods, physical activity events, or nonfood items for fundraising activities.
- Consider selling items such as produce, wrapping paper, candles, or student artwork.
- Organize events that engage students, families, and the community. Basketball or golf tournaments, bicycle rides, walk-a-thons, dance-a-thons, car washes, or auctions are healthy fundraising alternatives.

Create a Physically Active Classroom

Incorporate physical activity breaks in the classroom to help keep students focused and well-behaved.

- Incorporate movement into academic lessons or add short bursts of activity (5–20 minutes) to regularly planned break times.
- Read a book aloud while students walk at a moderate pace around the room, and then ask students to identify the verbs or action words in the book by acting them out through physical activity.
- Take students for a walk indoors or outdoors as part of a science lesson.
- Include content about fitness, movement skills and the importance of physical activity as part of math, science or writing lesson plans.

- Work with the physical education teacher to get ideas, information, and resources to help students stay physically active throughout the school day.

Make Recess Part of Each School Day

- Schedule at least 20 minutes of recess per day for elementary school students, in addition to their regularly scheduled physical education class.
- Encourage students to play during recess.
- Provide equipment, such as jump ropes and sports balls.
- Organize games, such as four-square, active tag, or flag football.
- Provide opportunities for students to be active indoors when the weather is bad or times when outdoor play space is unavailable.

Do Not Use Physical Activity as Punishment

Children may have negative feelings toward physical activity if they are forced to participate in physical activity as punishment. Further, withholding students from physical education or recess for bad behavior or poor academic performance deprives them of the health benefits of physical activity and the chance to develop essential physical activity skills. Physical education and recess may even improve students' behavior, attention, and test scores

- Do not punish students by forcing them to participate in or by withholding opportunities for physical activity.
- Do not punish students by requiring them to run laps or do push-ups.
- Do not exclude students from physical education class or recess.

Include Healthy Eating and Physical Activity Topics in Health Education

- Teach students about healthy eating and physical activity recommendations.

- Encourage students to participate in 60 minutes or more of physical activity every day, consume a healthy diet based on the Dietary Guidelines for Americans, 3 and reduce sedentary screen time (e.g., television, video games, computer usage).

- Encourage students to identify their own healthy behaviors and set personal goals for improvement.

- Incorporate health education into other subjects such as math and science.

- Extend healthy lessons outside of school by assigning homework for families to complete together.

- Meet with the school nurse to promote consistent health messages in your classroom. Consider asking the school nurse, or other health services staff, to lead a specific health lesson.

Watch Out for Student Weight Concerns and Stigma

- Address and intervene on all types of bullying, including weight discrimination and teasing about body shape or size.

- Refer students with signs of eating disorders, binge eating, or other weight concerns to the appropriate school staff such as the school nurse, counselor, psychologist, or school social worker.

Encourage Students to Participate in School Physical Activity Programs

- Support students in participating in intramural sport programs, interscholastic sports, physical activity clubs, or walk-and-bike to school programs.

- Promote school-led physical activity events, such as walk to school days, fun runs, and field days.
- Volunteer to organize or provide adult supervision to before and after school physical activity programs.

Be a Healthy Role Model

- Model healthy behaviors to students by being active and consuming healthy foods and beverages.
- Get involved in your school's employee wellness program or consider starting one. School wellness programs can include onsite opportunities for physical activity such as walking clubs, point-of-decision prompts that encourage use of stairwells, increased access to healthy foods, educational activities such as lectures or written materials, skill-building activities, or reward programs.

Become Familiar with Your School's Health Policies

- Read your district's local wellness policy and understand how the policy affects practices in your classroom.
- Get involved in your school health council or school health team. Suggest that the council or team assess healthy eating and physical activity policies and practices. If there is no school health council or school health team, consider starting one at your school by bringing together a variety of school staff, parents, and community members.

Source: *Tips for Teachers: Promoting Health Eating & Physical Activity in the Classroom.* Available at: http://www.cdc.gov/healthyyouth/npao/pdf/Tips_for_Teachers_TAG508.pdf.

Strategic Plan for NIH Obesity Research (2011)

The U.S. National Institutes of Health (NIH), the nation's medical research agency, conducts and supports research that provides scientific evidence for public policy decisions. The NIH encompasses

27 Institutes and Centers (ICs) and invests over $30 billion each through competitive grants to researchers in the United States and throughout the world.

To understand obesity research is the foundation for exploring the roles that genetics and biology, environment, and lifestyles play. Through research, it is possible to transform new knowledge into better prevention and treatment strategies, and to rigorously evaluate interventions to see which ones really work and who can benefit most. In April 2003, the NIH Obesity Research Task Force was formed to boost progress in obesity research. Key missions of the task force were to develop a strategic plan that would be a guide for coordinating obesity research activities across the NIH and to identify areas of greatest scientific opportunity and challenge. The resulting Strategic Plan for NIH Obesity Research emphasized the importance of interdisciplinary research teams to connect studies of behavioral and environmental causes of obesity with genetic and biologic causes. Disseminating research results to the public and health professionals was also the central component.

The 2004 plan called for research efforts along several fronts:

- *Behavioral and environmental approaches to modifying lifestyle to prevent or treat obesity*
- *Pharmacologic, surgical, and other medical approaches to effectively and safely prevent or treat obesity*
- *Breaking the link between obesity and diseases such as type 2 diabetes, heart disease, and certain cancers*
- *Research on special populations at high risk for obesity, including children, ethnic minorities, women, and older adults*
- *Translating basic science results into clinical research, and then into community intervention studies*

A new Strategic Plan for NIH Obesity Research published in 2011 enlarges the previous themes and encourages further investigations into the fresh opportunities, such as those presented by technology advances, which emerged in the years since the publication of NIH's first strategic plan. The plan incorporates the concepts that obesity arises from a complex interplay of forces and affects some populations disproportionately, and it is necessary take a multifaceted approach to combat it.

The 2011 strategic plan is framed around six new overarching research areas:

- *Discover fundamental biologic processes that regulate body weight and influence behavior*
- *Understand the factors that contribute to obesity and its consequences*
- *Design and test new interventions for achieving and maintaining a healthy weight*
- *Evaluate promising strategies for obesity prevention and treatment in real-world settings and diverse populations*
- *Harness technology and tools to advance obesity research and improve healthcare delivery*
- *Facilitate integration of research results into community programs and medical practice*

The excerpt below is a detailed description of the six areas of the 2011 Strategic Plan for NIH Obesity Research.

Research Opportunities

Research to identify and reduce health disparities is essential to all themes of the *Strategic Plan*. Populations at disproportionate risk for obesity include: racial and ethnic minority groups, such as African Americans, Hispanic/Latino Americans, American Indians/Alaska Natives, and Pacific Islanders; people who are socioeconomically disadvantaged and who have limited access to affordable healthy foods, safe places for physical activity, and health care; people with low literacy; and people who have physical, intellectual, or developmental disabilities.

Several additional topics span the themes of the *Strategic Plan*. An important area is translational research to bridge scientific discovery to improvements in public health: from fundamental insights gained in the laboratory into interventions that can be tested in clinical trials, and from results of clinical studies into research that explores implementation in real-world settings. A number of areas of NIH-supported obesity research may benefit from public-private partnerships and other collaborative efforts involving industries, schools, healthcare providers, community organizations, other government agencies, and other partners. Because obesity is increasing globally, studies in international settings may inform the development of prevention and treatment strategies for people around the world and in the United States. Finally, training and reinvigorating a multidisciplinary scientific workforce will be essential to the broad spectrum of research outlined in the *Strategic Plan*.

The following pages describe the major themes of the *Strategic Plan* in more detail. For each theme, the highlighted examples of research topics are intended to be illustrative, rather than limiting.

Discover Fundamental Biologic Processes That Regulate Body Weight and Influence Behavior

The extraordinary difficulties of preventing obesity, losing excess weight, and keeping the pounds off derive, in part, from the elaborate array of molecular signals that travel throughout the body to influence fat accumulation, eating behavior, and physical activity. The genes that encode these molecular signals vary from person to person: these genetic differences, which scientists are beginning to discover, make some people more, and others less, prone to obesity. Additionally, diet, activity, and aspects of our environment may modify innate biologic pathways in ways that increase, or protect against, excess body fat. By advancing knowledge of how body weight and metabolism are normally regulated, and what goes awry in obesity, fundamental research discoveries open new avenues for preventing and treating obesity and health problems related to excess weight. This research will identify factors that could be targeted by new drug development or other strategies, and it also will enhance the design of lifestyle interventions that more effectively address the biologic influences on people's behaviors.

Understand the Factors That Contribute to Obesity and Its Consequences

In addition to inherent biological factors, other potential contributors to excess weight gain include aspects of the environments in which we live; individual behaviors; and family, social, and cultural interactions. For example, the types and costs of foods available in communities, sedentary work and play, media and marketing messages that surround us, and local and national policies can all influence dietary choices and physical activity levels. Eating habits and physical activity also may change over time, and vary at different life stages in children and adults. Research to better understand the many factors that contribute to obesity, and how these differ among individuals and populations will provide insight into what could be changed to make environments and policies more conducive to healthy lifestyles, and to motivate and facilitate long-term behavior modification.

The consequences of obesity are numerous and varied. Obesity heightens the risk for type 2 diabetes, heart disease, many cancers, and a range of other serious and debilitating health conditions; impairs quality of life in other ways; and increases healthcare costs. Obesity may be both a cause and a consequence of other conditions, such as stress, sleep problems, depression, and binge eating disorder. Through research, increased knowledge of the consequences of obesity, how excess body fat can lead to disease, and how some people appear to stay healthy despite their obesity will facilitate development of more successful strategies to improve the health of all people who are obese.

Design and Test New Interventions for Achieving and Maintaining a Healthy Weight

Loss of even modest amounts of excess weight can have dramatic health benefits. Preventing obesity is associated with reduced risk for many serious diseases. However, the high rates of obesity in adults and children attest to the difficulty of achieving and maintaining a healthy weight. Thus, it will be important to design and evaluate a variety of obesity prevention and treatment approaches—both personalized and population-based. Examples include strategies to guide parents in providing healthy food and physical activity for their children; methods to help adults manage their own weight through healthier eating, increased exercise, and decreased sedentary activity; lifestyle interventions for achieving a healthy weight during pregnancy, to benefit mothers and their children; and approaches for maintaining healthy behaviors. These types of interventions can take place in a variety of settings—wherever people spend time, there are opportunities to promote a healthy lifestyle. Researchers can explore interventions in homes, schools, workplaces, healthcare settings, and other community sites. Researchers can also evaluate broader environmental and policy changes relevant to food and physical activity, to see which show promise. For people who are extremely obese or who already have an obesity-related illness, lifestyle approaches, although vital, may not be enough. Thus, continued studies of medications and surgical procedures will be valuable to help inform treatment decisions. It also will be important for researchers to determine whether weight control interventions reduce obesity-related diseases and improve quality of life.

*Evaluate Promising Strategies for Obesity Prevention
and Treatment in Real-World Settings and Diverse
Populations*

As we find successful approaches to prevent or reduce obesity, we can implement them more broadly, in healthcare practice and community settings, to benefit more people. Research will guide the development of cost-effective strategies to bring findings from clinical trials into real-world settings. In communities, research to evaluate new and existing policies and grassroots initiatives will spotlight those that show success and could be expanded. When an intervention seems promising, researchers can develop and test innovative adaptations for diverse populations and other settings where implementation may be more feasible or cost-effective. By surveying the landscape of obesity prevalence, neighborhood characteristics, and people's health and behaviors, researchers can identify populations that may have particular challenges to be addressed. Several avenues of study will yield information to help healthcare providers and their patients make decisions about weight management. This research includes comparing the outcomes of different lifestyle, pharmacologic, and surgical interventions, along with other forms of comparative effectiveness research. It is also important to ensure that weight control and related health information is communicated in meaningful ways. By exploring different communication strategies, researchers will improve ways to give people the health information they need, in terms they understand and that resonate with their own lives.

*Harness Technology and Tools to Advance Obesity
Research and Improve Healthcare Delivery*

Advances in technology and tools will bolster all of the research avenues described in the *Strategic Plan*, enhance delivery of health care, and improve people's ability to monitor their own diet and activity. Strategies to prevent and treat obesity would benefit from technologies to make a variety of measures feasible in real-world settings, more accurate, and cost-effective. These include measures of body fat, what and how much people are actually eating, how active or sedentary they are, and what types of foods and opportunities for physical activity are available in their neighborhoods. Advanced tools for collecting and analyzing very large amounts of data (high-throughput technologies) and other cutting-edge techniques will continue to accelerate research progress.

Facilitate Integration of Research Results into Community Programs and Medical Practice

To maximize the impact of research, the *Strategic Plan* highlights education, outreach, and other efforts to help community leaders, healthcare professionals, policymakers, and the general public make use of research findings. These include, for example, national education campaigns and programs for diverse audiences, such as an NIH education program to reduce childhood obesity called *We Can!*—Ways to Enhance Children's Activity & Nutrition. Additionally, the NIH has developed evidence-based clinical guidelines and other resources to help healthcare providers assist their patients with weight management. The NIH also collaborates and coordinates with other agencies and organizations to enhance research, patient care efforts, education, and outreach. These efforts will help educate the public, inform policy, and improve health care.

Source: NIH Obesity Research Task Force. *Strategic Plan for NIH Obesity Research*. NIH Publication No. 11–5493, March 2011. Available at: http://obesityresearch.nih.gov/about/StrategicPlanforNIH_Obesity_Research_Full-Report_2011.pdf.

Legislation

Regulation of Portion Sizes (2012)

The law shown here has an interesting story. In September 2012, New York City enacted a law to limit the maximum size of sugary beverages. Legislators hoped that this so-called "Portion Cap Rule" would reverse the super-size trend by restricting New Yorkers to smaller portion sizes and lead to reduction in consumption of sugary drinks and help control the increase in obesity. The law was to go into effect on March 16, 2013. The ban on these drinks was met with widespread controversy. Opponents argued that New York City was acting as a "nanny state" and infringing on individual rights. Others observed that the ban did not prevent an individual from just refilling an 8 ounce sugary beverage. On March 11, 2013, shortly before the law was to go into effect, the New York Supreme Court held that the ordinance was invalid, unconstitutional, and arbitrary, and capricious, and prohibited the city from enacting the Portion Cap Rule.

- Article 81: Food Preparation and Food Establishments

  Definition of terms used in this section.

  (1) *Sugary drink* means a carbonated or non-carbonated beverage that:

  (A) is non-alcoholic;

  (B) is sweetened by the manufacturer or establishment with sugar or another caloric sweetener;

  (C) has greater than 25 calories per 8 fluid ounces of beverage; and

  (D) does not contain more than 50 percent of milk or milk substitute by volume as an ingredient.

The volume of milk or milk substitute in a beverage will be presumed to be less than or equal to50 percent unless proven otherwise by the food service establishment serving it.

(2) *Milk substitute* means any liquid that is soy-based and is intended by its manufacturer to be a substitute for milk.

(3) *Self-service cup* means a cup or container provided by a food service establishment that is filled with a beverage by the customer.

(b) *Sugary drinks.* A food service establishment may not sell, offer, or provide a sugary drink in a cup or container that is able to contain more than 16 fluid ounces.

(c) *Self-service cups.* A food service establishment may not sell, offer, or provide to any customer a self-service cup or container that is able to contain more than 16 fluid ounces.

(d) *Violations of this section.* Notwithstanding the fines, penalties, and forfeitures outlined in Article 3 of this Code, a food service establishment determined to have violated this section will be subject to a fine of no more than two hundred dollars for each violation and no more than one violation of this section maybe cited at each inspection of a food service establishment.

Source: New York City Health Code, section 81.53. September 13, 2012. Available at: http://rules.cityofnewyork.us/content/section-8153-maximum-beverage-size.

Insurance Coverage for Obesity Prevention and Treatment (2013)

The dual purpose of this bill is to emphasize the problem of physical inactivity and poor eating habits in Idaho and to increase

*awareness of the role of registered dietitians (RDs) as the profes-
sional who can provide medical nutrition therapy (MNT) with a
focus on prevention and management of chronic conditions such
as obesity. MNT services are covered under Medicare, and federal
rules state that either RDs or other nutrition professionals may provide services if they meet certain education, experience, and certifi-
cation requirements. If individual states have a nutrition provider
licensure policy in place, then only the licensed individuals can
receive reimbursement. The legislation from Idaho recognizes dietitians but does not go as far as making them the exclusive MNT
providers.*

A CONCURRENT RESOLUTION STATING FINDINGS OF THE LEGISLATURE AND ENCOURAGING THE INCLUSION OF NUTRITION SERVICES AS AN INTEGRAL COMPONENT IN THE PREVENTION AND TREATMENT OF CHRONIC DISEASE

Be It Resolved by the Legislature of the State of Idaho:

WHEREAS, nearly 62% of Idaho's adult residents are overweight or obese due to poor nutrition and physical inactivity, putting them at risk for costly chronic diseases, such
as diabetes, heart disease and obesity-related cancers; and

WHEREAS, a reduction in the average Body Mass Index
(BMI) by five percent in Idaho's citizens could lead to
health care savings of more than one billion dollars in ten
years and three billion dollars in twenty years; and

WHEREAS, nutrition and wellness classes provided by
registered dietitians have resulted in positive outcomes
in BMI, blood sugars and reduction of heart disease risk
throughout Idaho; and

WHEREAS, registered dietitians in Idaho collaborate with
other medical professionals to deliver Medical Nutrition
Therapy (MNT), ensuring a patient's overall health with
an emphasis on prevention, improved clinical outcomes
and reducing health care costs; and

WHEREAS, according to the Institute of Medicine, "the registered dietitian is currently the single identifiable group of health-care professionals with standardized education, clinical training, continuing education and national credentialing requirements necessary to be directly reimbursed as a provider of nutrition therapy"; and

WHEREAS, registered dietitians work in a variety of professions and locations throughout Idaho in the private and public sector and are trained medical professionals who are licensed through the Idaho State Board of Medicine.

NOW, THEREFORE, BE IT RESOLVED by the members of the First Regular Session of the Sixty-second Idaho Legislature, the House of Representatives and the Senate concurring therein, that the Legislature finds that registered dietitians can help the people of Idaho in the selection of nutritious foods, including Idaho food products, prevent and manage diseases through MNT and counseling, and provide nutrition education in schools, workplaces, clinics and other venues.

BE IT FURTHER RESOLVED that by providing MNT and professional nutrition counseling by Idaho registered dietitians in conjunction with existing services covered by insurance carriers, there will be a significant impact on chronic disease management, along with significant health care cost savings in the State of Idaho.

Source: Legislature of the State of Idaho, House Concurrent Resolution 19 (2013). 62nd Legislature, ID HCR 19 (2013). Available at: http://www.legislature.idaho.gov/legisla tion/2013/HCR019.pdf.

Ensuring Healthy Food in Schools (2013)

This bill makes changes to bring California's school cafeteria and nutrition laws into compliance with changes in federal nutrition regulations that require schools to serve food options that align with healthful meal patterns. As part of a larger law, this section

describes which beverages are considered to be "nonnutritious" and defines regulations for restricting sales and access to them in schools. In contrast to the previous variety of food and beverages eligible for sale, this measure specifies that only food and beverage items that meet the state and federal nutrition standards may be sold from 30 minutes before the start of the school day until 30 minutes after the end of the school day.

SEC. 4.

Section 35182.5

(a) The Legislature finds and declares all of the following:

(1) State and federal laws require all schools participating in meal programs to provide nutritious food and beverages to pupils.

(2) State and federal laws restrict the sale of food and beverages in competition with meal programs to enhance the nutritional goals for pupils, and to protect the fiscal and nutritional integrity of the school food service programs.

(3) Parents, pupils, and community members should have the opportunity to ensure, through the review of food and beverage contracts, that food and beverages sold on school campuses provide nutritious sustenance to pupils, promote good health, help pupils learn, provide energy, and model fit living for life.

(b) For purposes of this section, the following terms have the following meanings:

(1) "Nonnutritious beverages" means any beverage that is not any of the following:

(A) Drinking water.

(B) Milk, including, but not limited to, chocolate milk, soy milk, rice milk, and other similar dairy or nondairy milk.

(C) An electrolyte replacement beverage that contains 42 grams or less of added sweetener per 20 ounce serving.

(D) A 100 percent fruit juice, or fruit-based drink that is composed of 50 percent or more fruit juice and that has no added sweeteners.

(2) "Added sweetener" means any additive that enhances the sweetness of the beverage, including, but not limited to, added sugar, but does not include the natural sugar or sugars that are contained within any fruit juice that is a component of the beverage.

(3) "Nonnutritious food" means food that is not sold as part of the school breakfast or lunch program as a full meal, and that meets any of the following standards:

(A) More than 35 percent of its total calories are from fat.

(B) More than 10 percent of its total calories are from saturated fat.

(C) More than 35 percent of its total weight is composed of sugar. This subparagraph does not apply to the sale of fruits or vegetables.

SEC. 9.

Section 49431

(a) (1) From one-half hour before the start of the schoolday to one-half hour after the schoolday, at each elementary school, the only food that may be sold to a pupil are full meals, individually sold dairy or whole grain foods, and individually sold portions of nuts, nut butters, seeds, eggs, cheese packaged for individual sale, fruit, vegetables that have not been deep fried, and legumes.

(2) An individually sold dairy or whole grain food item, and individually sold portions of nuts, nut butters,

seeds, eggs, cheese packaged for individual sale, fruit, vegetables that have not been deep fried, and legumes may be sold to pupils at an elementary school, except food sold as part of a USDA meal program, if they meet all of the following standards:

(A) Not more than 35 percent of its total calories shall be from fat. This subparagraph shall not apply to individually sold portions of nuts, nut butters, seeds, eggs, cheese packaged for individual sale, fruit, vegetables that have not been deep fried, or legumes.

(B) Not more than 10 percent of its total calories shall be from saturated fat. This subparagraph shall not apply to eggs or cheese packaged for individual sale.

(C) Not more than 35 percent of its total weight shall be composed of sugar, including naturally occurring and added sugar. This subparagraph shall not apply to fruit or vegetables that have not been deep fried.

(D) Not more than 175 calories per individual food item.

(b) An elementary school may permit the sale of food items that do not comply with subdivision (a) as part of a school fundraising event in either of the following circumstances:

(1) The sale of those items takes place off of and away from school premises.

(2) The sale of those items takes place on school premises at least one-half hour after the end of the schoolday.

(c) It is the intent of the Legislature that the governing board of a school district annually review its compliance with the nutrition standards described in this section and Section 49431.5.

SEC. 10.

[similar restrictions are listed for middle and high schools]

SEC. 11.

Section 49431.5

(a) (1) Regardless of the time of day, only the following beverages may be sold to a pupil at an elementary school:

(A) Fruit-based drinks that are composed of no less than 50 percent fruit juice and have no added sweetener.

(B) Vegetable-based drinks that are composed of no less than 50 percent vegetable juice and have no added sweetener.

(C) Drinking water with no added sweetener.

(D) One-percent-fat milk, nonfat milk, soy milk, rice milk, and other similar nondairy milk.

(2) An elementary school may permit the sale of beverages that do not comply with paragraph (1) as part of a school fundraising event in either of the following circumstances:

(A) The sale of those items takes place off and away from the premises of the school.

(B) The sale of those items takes place on school premises at least one-half hour after the end of the schoolday.

(3) From one-half hour before the start of the schoolday to one-half hour after the end of the schoolday, only the following beverages may be sold to a pupil at a middle school or high school:

(A) Fruit-based drinks that are composed of no less than 50 percent fruit juice and have no added sweetener.

(B) Vegetable-based drinks that are composed of no less than 50 percent vegetable juice and have no added sweetener.

(C) Drinking water with no added sweetener.

(D) One-percent-fat milk, nonfat milk, soy milk, rice milk, and other similar nondairy milk.

(E) An electrolyte replacement beverage that contains no more than 42 grams of added sweetener per 20-ounce serving.

(4) A middle school or high school may permit the sale of beverages that do not comply with paragraph (3) as part of a school event if the sale of those items meets either of the following criteria:

(A) The sale of those items takes place off and away from the premises of the school.

(B) The sale of those items takes place on school premises at least one-half hour after the end of the schoolday.

Source: California Assembly Bill 626. School Nutrition. Approved October 10, 2013. Available at: http://leginfo.legislature .ca.gov/faces/billNavClient.xhtml?bill_id=201320140AB626.

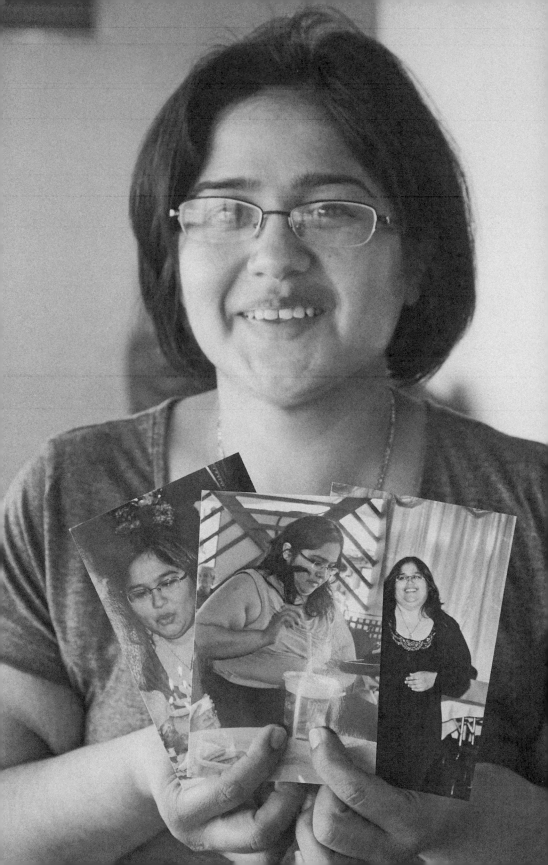

There are many resources available to help you get more information about obesity. These specific resources include those from government agencies, nonprofit organizations, scientific experts, newspapers, magazines, popular authors, and entrepreneurs. This list is not all inclusive. It highlights some important resources that will allow the reader to see the range of information that is available on topics related to obesity and to explore those in more depth.

Books

Reference Books

Handbook of Obesity, Two-Volume Set: Fourth Edition

George A Bray, Claude Bouchard, Editors
CRC Press, 2014. 528 p.
ISBN: 978–1841849812

This two-volume set is comprised of the 3rd edition of Volume 1 and the 4th edition of Volume 2. Presenting the

A woman shows off "before" photographs after undergoing a robotic kidney transplant, obesity surgery, and regular workouts at her local YMCA. Whether it is information about bariatric surgery, methods to reduce calories and increase physical activity, basic metabolism and physiology, or dietary supplements, meal plans, and recipes, there are hundreds of resources about obesity. New research and clinical techniques are reported each day online and in the popular and scientific press. (AP Photo/M. Spencer Green)

insight of international experts and edited by two eminent leaders in obesity research, this edition reflects the evolving understanding of obesity. It is a comprehensive and up-to-date guide for healthcare providers to diagnose and treat obese patients. Volume One: "Epidemiology, Etiology, and Physiopathology" provides comprehensive coverage of the biological, behavioral, and environmental determinants of obesity. Some sections included are the history and changes over time that surrounds our notion of obesity and the epidemiology of obesity in various populations. Volume Two: "Clinical Applications" explores essential factors involved in obesity prevention and treatment including strategies for evaluation of patients with overweight or obesity as well as current medical treatments and surgeries.

Practical Manual of Clinical Obesity

Robert Kushner, Victor Lawrence, and Sudhesh Kumar

Wiley-Blackwell, 2013. 204pp.

ISBN: 978–0470654767

This manual provides clinically focused guidance for healthcare professionals involved in the treatment of patients with obesity. The chapters contain features such as key points, pitfall boxes, management flowcharts, and case studies to enable a broad understanding of obesity diagnosis and management. Key clinical trials and major international society guidelines are referred to throughout. This book provides accessible information for health professionals of all levels who manage obese patients, such as nurses, dietitians, and general practitioners.

Popular Books

The listing of a popular book does not mean that it is an approved book or approved diet. Check the Federal Trade Commission report entitled "Weight Loss Advertising" in the Reports section of this chapter to see the criteria for appraising the value of diets and claims.

The Alternative Day Diet Revised

James B. Johnson and Donald Laub

Perigee Trade, 2013. 288pp.

ISBN: 978–0399167034

This is an updated and expanded version of the original intermittent fasting diet, *The Alternative Day Diet: Diet Only Half the Time*. The diet plan is a modified fast. On the "down days," dieters must limit themselves to 300–500 calories. For the down days in the first few weeks, dieters are advised to sip protein shakes throughout the day. On other days, there are no foods that are off limits. The revised edition contains additional techniques, including supplementation and eating according to the body's natural circadian rhythms to enhance the diet's effectiveness. Both authors are plastic surgeons.

Don't Eat This Book: Fast Food and the Supersizing of America

Morgan Spurlock

The Penguin Group, 2005. 320pp.

ISBN: 0399152601

After filming his movie *Supersize Me*, Morgan Spurlock wrote this book to further support the conclusions of his 30-day Mc-Donald's Diet and he explains why he believes so many Americans are obese today. In this book, he discusses interviews he held with law officials, marketing professionals, and obesity experts.

Fast Food Nation

Eric Schlosser

HarperCollins Publishers, 2002. 416pp.

ISBN: 978–0547750330

Journalist Schlosser, in *Fast Food Nation*, takes an inside look at the fast-food industry. He has been investigating the fast-food industry for years and he discusses what he has found in great detail in this book, including how it has created the obesity epidemic, insight on how the food is prepared and produced, and how the industry targets our younger population through advertising. Some of the chapters are: "Why the Fries Taste So Good," "On the Range," and "What's in the Meat?" In 2006, this book was adapted into a movie of the same name.

Fat Land: How Americans Became the Fattest People in the World

Greg Critser
Houghton Mifflin Company, 2002. 256pp.
ISBN: 0618164723

Greg Critser explains how so many Americans became obese, using examples of differences in class, politics, culture, and economics. As a person who has been overweight in the past, he is able to provide an inside look at the challenges associated with being overweight. Chapters included are: "Supersize Me," "What the Extra Calories Do to You," and "What Can Be Done."

Fit from the Start: How to Prevent Childhood Obesity in Infancy

Alvin N. Eden, Barbara J. Moore, and Adrienne Forman
Shape Up America!, 2014. 143pp.
ISBN: 0991530225

This book is based on the concept that obesity prevention begins the day a child is born. While obesity has a built-in genetic component, it may be possible to control expression of those genes through healthful eating and exercise. The authors include a pediatrician, a scientist, and a nutritionist who explain the importance of family diet and activity choices for infants, children, and also the parents and caregivers. The book contains practical tips, including when to introduce infants to solid food, how babies who do not walk can still be active, and how all family members can take part in an enjoyable lifestyle that may prevent obesity.

Food Fight

Kelly D. Brownell and Katherine B. Horgen, PhD.
McGraw-Hill Companies, 2004. 356pp.
ISBN: 978–0071438728

This book looks at how we live in a "toxic environment" when it comes to dietary health. It explores the factors that have created an increase in disease and an expanded waistline in America. *Food Fight* includes the authors' explanation of how the "toxic environment" was created, what fuels it in our society, and what steps need to be taken to combat it.

Food Politics: How the Food Industry Influences Nutrition and Health, Revised and Expanded Edition

Marion Nestle
University of California Press, 2007. 457pp.
ISBN: 978–0520224650

Food Politics, written by NYU's Professor Marion Nestle, takes an inside look at how the main goal of food companies is to sell more product by encouraging us to eat more. The abundance of food in the United States—enough calories to meet the needs of every man, woman, and child twice over—has a downside. Dr. Nestle describes how the mass production and consumption of food is driven by economics instead of science, common sense, or health.

Food Rules: An Eater's Manual

Michael Pollan
Penguin Books, 2009. 140pp.
ISBN: 978–0143116387

This small book has been called "A definitive compendium of food wisdom."

Michael Pollan asserts that eating does not have to be complicated. He lays out a set of straightforward rules for eating wisely, one per page, accompanied by a concise explanation. His principles are drawn from a variety of traditions, suggesting how different cultures through the ages have arrived at the same enduring wisdom about food.

Mayo Clinic Healthy Weight for Everybody
Mayo Clinic, 2005. 240pp.
ISBN: 978–1893005341

This is a comprehensive, quick reference guide from the world renowned Mayo Clinic that provides the tools to get started with an individual weight loss and maintenance program. Features include a full color insert featuring delicious recipes; tips on shopping smarter; advice on how to maintain weight loss; and detailed strategies for devising a fitness plan.

Mindless Eating: Why We Eat More Than We Think
Brian Wansink
Bantam Dell, 2006. 276pp.
ISBN: 978–0553384482

Brian Wansink is a Professor at Cornell University who has spent time at USDA. *Mindless Eating* examines the variables that cause one to consume food. Topics include food marketing and other environmental cues that influence our eating behavior, experiments he and his students have conducted that look at how we make dietary decisions, and how to "Mindlessly Eat Better."

Tyler's Honest Herbal, 4th Edition
Steven Foster and Varro E. Tyler
Haworth Press, 1999. 442pp.
ISBN: 0789007053

A number of dietary supplements for weight loss contain herbs or herbal extracts. *The Honest Herbal* was originally published in the late 1970s. It continues to be a frequently referenced, quoted, and controversial book on herbs. Varro Tyler is a distinguished professor emeritus at Purdue University. In the preface, the authors write that herbs can make a significant positive contribution to health, but a scientific point-of-view is crucial. In terms of weight loss, the discussion about *Garcinia* is an excellent example of how the authors reviewed the evidence. A number of studies in lean and obese rats found that hydroxycitrate is a primary acid found in *Garcini cambogia*. The authors concluded that, while there are a number of studies in obese rats, "the effects of garcinia preparations on obese humans are noticeably absent from the literature . . . new studies are need before garcinia. . . .can be considered useful for controlling obesity in humans . . . garcinia products have successfully lightened the bank accounts of consumers."

The Volumetrics Eating Plan: Techniques and Recipes for Feeling Full on Fewer Calories

Barbara J. Rolls
Harper Collins, 2005. 317pp.
ISBN: 978–0060737306

The Volumetrics Eating Plan by Professor and Researcher Barbara J. Rolls provides strategies and easy-to-prepare recipes to encourage eating foods that are low in energy density. Those foods—fruits, vegetables, and soups—are all high in water content and low in energy density. These foods tend to be more filling, so one eats fewer calories even while getting a larger volume of food. The emphasis is on developing lifelong healthy eating skills. Rolls is an internationally known researcher on food intake and weight management.

Why We Get Fat: And What to Do About It

Gary Taubes
Alfred A. Knopf, 2010. 272pp.
ISBN: 0307474259

Science journalist Taubes updates his 2007 book *Good Calories, Bad Calories: Challenging the Conventional Wisdom on Diet, Weight Control, and Disease.* This book contains his explanation of the dangers of dietary carbohydrates. He asks, "If the USDA dietary guidelines recommending that highly caloric grains and carbohydrates comprise 45 to 65 percent of daily caloric intake are so healthy, why has obesity among Americans been on the upswing? Why has this same diet, endorsed by the American Heart Association, not managed to reduce the incidence of heart disease?" Taubes describes some science that discredits the idea that weight control is a simple matter of burning more calories than one consumes and he offers an alternative viewpoint: no carbohydrates. His recommendation for weight management and health is to eliminate carbohydrates (grains, fruits, and sugars) from one's diet.

Reports

Comprehensive Report on 2000 Growth Charts

Series Report 11, Number 246. 2000, 201pp.
PHS 2001–1695.
Web site: http://www.cdc.gov/nchs/data/series/sr_11/sr11 _246.pdf.

This comprehensive report, from the U.S. Centers for Disease Control and Prevention (CDC), includes the 2000 CDC pediatric growth charts for boys and girls ranging in age from 2 to 20 years old. The charts were developed by the National Center for Health Statistics 1977 and revised in 2000. Most of these data came from the National Health and Nutrition

Evaluation Survey (NHANES). These charts are used by healthcare workers to assess growth of infants, children, and adolescents in the United States. The 1977 charts were adopted for international use by the WHO.

Deception in Weight Loss Advertising

R. L. Cleland, W. C. Gross, L. D. Koss, M. Daynard, K. M. Muolo

Federal Trade Commission, 2002, pp40 + Appendix
Web site: https://www.ftc.gov/sites/default/files/documents/reports/deception-weight-loss-advertising-workshop-seizing-opportunities-and-building-partnerships-stop/031209weight-lossrpt.pdf.

This was an important report released in 2002 by the FTC with the Partnership for Healthy Weight Management (a coalition of representatives from science, academia, heath care professions, government, commercial enterprises, and organizations), whose mission is to promote sound guidance on strategies for achieving and maintaining a healthy weight. The findings of the FTC indicate that by improving Americans' health literacy they can have information they need to make appropriate health decisions. It encourages the media to undertake a role in educating consumers by providing accurate information about weight loss programs and weight management products.

Dietary Reference Intakes: The Essential Guide to Nutrient Requirements

J. M. McGinnis (Chair)
The National Academies Press, 2006, 560pp.
ISBN: 0309100917
Web site: http://www.nap.edu/openbook.php?record_id=11537&page=R3.

This report from the National Academies of Sciences is a summary of eight volumes in one reference volume. It is organized by nutrient and reviews the function of each nutrient, its food sources, and recommendations for people for maintenance of health and reduction of risk of chronic diseases such as CVD and some cancers. It breaks out estimated average requirements by sex and age. It also gives estimates as to tolerable upper levels to avoid toxicity of some nutrients.

Food Marketing to Children: Threat or Opportunity

J.M. McGinnis, J.A. Gootman, V.I. Kraak (Editors)

National Academies of Sciences Press, 2005, 536pp.

ISBN: 978–0309097130

Web site: https://www.iom.edu/Reports/2005/Food-Market ing-to-Children-and-Youth-Threat-or-Opportunity.aspx.

This report, requested by the U.S. Congress and produced by the CDC, is a comprehensive review of the impact of food marketing on nutritional beliefs, choices, practices, and outcomes for children and youth. The authors conclude that many of these advertised products targeted to young people are high in calories, fat, and sugar, and so they are out of balance with recommendations for a healthful diet. Additionally, the report finds that policies intended to control advertisements often do not have the support needed to regulate marketing practices that have an important influence on the desired food choices of children and youth.

Gut Check: A Reference Guide for Media on Spotting False Weight Loss Claims

Federal Trade Commission

Web site: https://www.ftc.gov/tips-advice/business-center/ guidance/gut-check-reference-guide-media-spotting-false- weight-loss.

With this guide, the FTC, our nation's consumer protection agency, describes how to identify false weight loss claims. The guide is intended for broadcasters and publishers to screen advertisements before they are accepted for publication or airing. A checklist of seven weight loss claims that could not possibly be true (e.g., a product will cause weight loss no matter what or how much a person eats) is provided, so editors can do a "gut check"—or to look with some skepticism at such ads to spot any tip-offs to deceptive product promotions.

Preventing Childhood Obesity: Health in the Balance

J. P. Koplan, C. T. Liverman, V. A. Kraak (Editors)
The National Academies Press, 2005, 436pp.
ISBN: 0309091969
Web site: http://www.iom.edu/Reports/2004/Preventing-Childhood-Obesity-Health-in-the-Balance.aspx.

This committee report from the National Academy of Sciences examines the environmental, social, medical, and historic factors influencing childhood obesity. Most dramatic is the statement that "The increased number of obese children throughout the U.S. during the past 25 years has led policymakers to rate it as one of the most critical public health threats of the 21st-century." The report includes recommendations to help mobilize parents to find solutions to this important problem, which includes identification of short-term and longer term interventions.

School Policy Framework: Implementation of the WHO Global Strategy on Diet, Physical Activity and Health

WHO Consultation on Obesity, World Health Organization, Geneva, 2008, pp276.
ISBN: 978–9241596862

Because healthy children can achieve better educational outcomes, the World Health Organization (WHO) developed a framework or a practical tool that promotes healthful food and activity opportunities for school children throughout the world. The framework is intended to be a guide for individual countries, both developed and developing, to set national policies such as those that could improve physical activity and fitness and to increase children's consumption of fruits and vegetables.

Strategic Plan for NIH Obesity Research

National Institutes of Health (NIH), 2011.

NIH publication N. 04–5493

Web site: http://obesityresearch.nih.gov/about/strategic-plan.aspx.

This report was originally published in 2004 as a guide for co-ordinating obesity research at NIH and for enhancing research in areas of greatest scientific opportunity. The new 2011 *Strategic Plan for NIH Obesity Research* serves as a guide to encourage and accelerate a wide range of research aimed toward developing new and more effective approaches to address the burden of obesity. This updated *Strategic Plan* reflects the opportunities that have emerged in the years since the publication of the first plan for research. New research challenges and opportunities, identified at a variety of meetings and workshops, continue to inform NIH research planning. More information about the plan is in the Data and Documents chapter of this book.

The State of Obesity

J. Levi, L. M. Segal, R. St. Laurent, A. Lang, J. Rayburn

Trust for America's Health

Web site: http://stateofobesity.org/.

Since 2004, an annual report, *The State of Obesity* (formerly *F as in Fat*), has raised awareness about the seriousness of the obesity epidemic, encouraged the creation of a national obesity prevention strategy, and highlighted promising approaches for reversing the epidemic at the state and local level. The report is a collaborative project of the Trust for America's Health and the Robert Wood Johnson Foundation. After 10 years of being titled *F as in Fat*, the report became *The State of Obesity: Better Policies for a Healthier America*. The authors believe the "F" no longer needs to stand for failure. The new approach is to identify the "state of obesity" in America today as there are successes as well as continuing failures. For example, the 2014 report shows signs of progress in that, after decades of increases, childhood obesity rates have stabilized in the past decade.

Guidelines

Aim for a Healthy Weight

The National Heart, Lung, and Blood Institute (NHLBI)
Publication No. 05–5213
Web site: http://www.nhlbi.nih.gov/health/public/heart/obesity/aim_hwt.htm.

This booklet provides a step-by-step guide to develop a personal food and exercise plan. There are numerous tables and lists of common sense hints that present the basics such as how to determine BMI and how it is related to health. A "Healthy Eating Plan" describes how to reduce calories by being aware of portion sizes, cooking methods, and ideas for substitutes for high-calorie foods. There are hints for types of fast foods to choose to stay within weight reduction guidelines and a section on types of physical activities and the number of calories that can be burned for each. This is a good all-in-one starter's guide for weight management.

2008 Physical Activity Guidelines for Americans

Office of Disease Prevention and Health Promotion
Web site: http://www.health.gov/paguidelines/guidelines/.

There were no federal physical activity guidelines reported before 2008 because the Department of Health and Human Services experts questioned whether there was enough data to support any specific recommendations. This report was the result of workshops with scientists, physical activity practitioners, and government agencies. The consensus was that physical activity significantly contributes to health and that public health programs would benefit from some guidelines to set their agendas. These guidelines describe daily and weekly goals for various population groups and physical conditions. The report was released in collaboration with the Dietary Guidelines Committee, as food and activity must both be considered when setting health objectives.

Guidelines for Managing Overweight and Obesity in Adults, 2013

American Heart Association, American College of Cardiology, The Obesity Society (AHA/ACC/TOS)

Web site: http://circ.ahajournals.org/content/early/2013/11/11/01.cir.0000437739.71477.ee.

The 2013 *Guidelines* summarizes the research that occurred since the first 1998 guidelines were reported, and included updated knowledge about interventions for weight loss and weight loss maintenance. There are new recommendations concerning surgeries and medications. The overall message in the new report is that any weight management program should be customized for each person as there are no broad plans that work for everyone. The plans should include methods to reduce calories, increase physical activity, and provide personalized behavior strategies to help individuals reach and maintain a healthy weight.

Dietary Guidelines for Americans, 2010

DHHS and USDA
USDA Center for Nutrition Policy and Promotion

Web site: http://www.health.gov/dietaryguidelines/dga2010/ DietaryGuidelines2010.pdf.

The U.S. dietary guidelines are revised every five years. This was the 2010 edition that was developed after examining new research about food, activity, and health outcomes that appeared after the *2005 Dietary Guidelines*. One of the nine focus areas in this report was "maintaining a healthy weight." There are no exact recommendations about how to reduce weight. The *Guidelines* support a generally healthy diet that could be used by anyone. But suggested foods such as those low in fat, low in calories, and higher in fiber are components of many weight control diet plans. The MyPlate eating plan appeared in the *Guidelines* this year, replacing the commonly maligned MyPyramid.

Healthy People 2010

Web site: healthypeople.gov

The goal of *Healthy People 2020* (HP2020) is to provide a guide for improving the health of all Americans. Based on science and advances in medicine and disease surveillance, the mission of HP2020 is to identify health improvement priorities for the next decade, increase public awareness about the priorities, and support research in those areas. An overarching aim of HP2020 is to achieve health equity and eliminate disparities for all groups regardless of age, gender identification, ethnicity, or economic status. The initiative also provides measurable goals that are assessed at the local, state, and national levels. About halfway through the 10-year period, the goals are evaluated and used as a basis to set new aims for the subsequent HP plan. The entire initiative is also assessed at the end of the decade to determine and report on how, and if, goals were met.

Healthy People 2020

Web site: http://www.healthypeople.gov.

Healthy People 2020 is based on the accomplishments of four previous decades of Healthy People programs. It was released in 2010 as the nation's 10-year goals and objectives for health promotion and disease prevention. Along with the new goals, HHS also launched a redesigned *Healthy People* Web site and *Healthy People eLearning*, an online educational resource designed to help students and health professionals learn how to reach these health goals.

School Health Guidelines

Web site: http://www.cdc.gov/healthyyouth/npao/strate gies.htm.

In 2011, the U.S. Centers for Disease Control released *School Health Guidelines to Promote Healthy Eating and Physical Activity*, a report synthesized from up-to-date scientific evidence and best practices by education professionals. The guidelines incorporate the 2010 *Dietary Guidelines for Americans*, the 2008 *Physical Activity Guidelines for Americans*, and the *Healthy People 2020* objectives to provide nine areas that serve as the foundation for developing, implementing, and evaluating school-based healthy eating and physical activity policies and practices for students in grades K–12. Each of the nine guidelines is accompanied by specific strategies for schools to put into action.

Journals and Magazines

These are examples of periodicals that have up-to-date information about many aspects of obesity and weight management.

Consumer Reports

Publisher: Consumers Union
ISSN: 0010–7174
Web site: http://www.consumerreports.org.

Consumer Reports is published monthly by Consumers Union, a nonprofit, independent testing and information organization. It does not accept advertisements to maintain its independence and to be a reliable source of information. *Consumer Reports* has reviewed weight loss supplements and diets and diet programs. A 2013 *Consumer Reports* article describes their survey of 9,736 people about the diets they tried. The authors rated 13 popular diets. Most of them, like the Atkins Diet and the South Beach Diet, are do-it-yourself as all that is usually needed are instructions from a book or Web site, in some cases, a computer app. The results of the study are presented in an interesting way as the diets are arranged by who the diet is best for. Some examples are the Atkins Diet that is best for people who love the idea of a diet that lets them eat bacon, steak, and full-fat mayonnaise. Jenny Craig is best for dieters who hate cooking and have trouble with portion control and Weight Watchers is best for people who appreciate support.

International Journal of Obesity

Publisher: Nature Publishing Group, Inc.

ISSN: 0307–0565

Web site: http://www.nature.com/ijo/index.html.

International Journal of Obesity is the official research journal of the International Association for the Study of Obesity. It is published monthly. It publishes research papers on basic, clinical, and applied studies that address the biochemical, genetic, nutritional, psychological, and sociological aspects of obesity.

Journal of the Academy of Nutrition and Dietetics

Publisher: Elsevier

ISSN: 2212–2672

Web site: http://www.journals.elsevier.com/journal-of-the-academy-of-nutrition-and-dietetics/.

The *Journal of the Academy of Nutrition and Dietetics* was formerly titled the *Journal of the American Dietetic*

Association until January 2012 when the Academy underwent an organization-wide name change. Registered dietitian nutritionists rely on the *Journal* as a source of peer-reviewed articles, position papers, and topics of current interest.

New England Journal of Medicine

Publisher: Massachusetts Medical Society
ISSN: 0028–4793
Web site: http://www.nejm.org/.

The *New England Journal of Medicine* is published weekly and is the official journal of the Massachusetts Medical Society. It publishes individual research articles, review articles, and commentaries. The articles are targeted to physicians and other healthcare professionals, and are dedicated to presenting the information in an understandable and clinically useful format, and to keeping practitioners connected to both clinical science and the values of being a good physician. It is one of the important sources of medical news.

Nutrition Today

Publisher: Wolters Kluwer Health, Inc.
ISSN: 0029–666X
Web site: http://journals.lww.com/nutritiontodayonline/pages/default.aspx.

Nutrition Today, the partner publication of the *American Society for Nutrition*, is published six times a year. It is primarily for nutritional professionals, but it is easy-to-read and valuable to consumers who are interested in wide-ranging nutrition topics, from sports nutrition to the food business to leading nutrition and health professionals' opinions about the politics of food.

Obesity

Publisher: Wiley-Blackwell
ISSN: 1930–739X
Web site: http://www.obesity.org/publications/obesity-journal.htm.

Obesity (formerly known as *Obesity Research*) is the official journal of The Obesity Society. It publishes research and review articles, commentaries, public health and medical developments, and abstracts from its annual meeting. *Obesity* features a front section to help readers stay abreast of the latest information. This section includes editorials, commentaries, and timely and relevant coverage of research that defines the field. It is published monthly.

Obesity Facts

The European Journal of Obesity
Publisher: Karger
ISSN: 1662–4025
Web site: www.karger.com/OFA.

Obesity Facts, first published in 2008, is the official journal of the European Association for the Study of Obesity. The editors aim to report recent research findings on obesity that cover a broad area of interest such as the impact of nutrition and exercise, psychological and sociological factors, and diseases that are comorbidities of obesity. The journal is targeted to all healthcare professionals concerned with obesity issues. For example, a diverse population that includes pediatricians, sports medicine specialists, sociologists, biologists, and public health researchers will find the latest scientific developments in their respective fields.

Obesity Reviews

Publisher: Wiley-Blackwell

ISSN: 1467–789X

Web site: http://onlinelibrary.wiley.com/journal/10.1111/%28ISSN%291467–789X.

Obesity Reviews is a monthly journal publishing reviews on all disciplines related to obesity and its comorbidities. This includes basic and behavioral sciences, clinical treatment and outcomes, epidemiology, prevention, and public health. *Obesity Reviews* is the official journal of the World Obesity Federation, which links over 50 regional and national associations with more than 10,000 professional members. Many reviews are available for free on the Web site. Examples of the 2015 reviews include: "Outcomes of Bariatric Surgery" and "From Genetics, Epigenetics, and Prevention to Management." The journal also publishes free access to articles that debate key topics in obesity with pro versus con reviews such as: "Food industry: friend or foe?"; "Role of sugar sweetened beverages in obesity,"; and "Is Food Addictive?"

Web Sites

General Population Information and Interactive Sites

ChooseMyPlate.gov

Web site: http://www.choosemyplate.gov/en-espanol.html.

Launched in 2011, *MyPlate* is a colorful visual of a meal place setting that shows how to make healthful food choices by providing an example of portion sizes for different food groups. Consumers can use the plate icon to estimate the relative amounts of fruit, vegetable, grains, protein foods, and dairy groups that make up a healthful diet. A key message is that half the plate and half the foods one eats should be fruits and vegetables. In addition to the plate as a guide, there are numerous online tools and practical information to help make *MyPlate* part of a daily diet. "Your daily food plan" specifies how many servings of fruits, vegetables, protein, grains, and dairy a person needs based on age, weight, and height. To track daily calories and physical activity, a link to the *SuperTracker* site is included. *ChooseMyPlate.gov* provides educational material presented as quizzes such as: "Name that Veggie" and "Test Your Salt Savvy." The user-friendly Web site is geared toward all Americans and is a valuable resource for health and food industry professionals as well as consumers. In addition to English, Spanish, Chinese, Hindi, Japanese, Urdu, and Vietnamese are a few of the languages in which *MyPlate* is available.

FDA Dietary Supplements

Web site: http://www.fda.gov/Food/DietarySupplements/default.htm.

People trying to lose weight may turn to over-the-counter dietary weight loss supplements, as the products promise easy ways to reduce body fat. Supplements are attractive because they are often marketed as "natural," which may be interpreted that they are safe and effective. It is the responsibility of the Food and Drug Administration (FDA) to regulate dietary supplements, using a set of regulations set forth by the Dietary Supplement Health and Education Act, which are different from those covering foods and drugs. While it seems that actual occurrences of FDA regulation are sparse, this Web site does provide information to help consumers to decide for themselves about whether supplements could be helpful, harmful, or have no effect. The site also includes answers to frequently asked questions such as: What exactly is a dietary supplement, and what does it mean when a label states, "This statement has not been evaluated by the FDA. This product is not intended to diagnose, treat, cure, or prevent any disease"?

Consumers can also report a complaint or adverse event concerning a nutrition supplement here.

Health at Every Size

Web site: http://www.haescommunity.org/.

This is the companion Web site for *Health at Every Size: The Surprising Truth About Your Weight* by Linda Bacon. The *Health at Every Size* premise is acknowledgment that good health can best be realized independent from considerations of size. It supports people of all sizes in addressing health directly by adopting healthy behaviors. The site provides links to resources such as HAES-friendly products and providers. To show commitment to HAES, Web site readers are encouraged to sign the HAES Pledge with the ideas that as word spreads, institutional change may be hastened by demonstrating that there is a large audience for HAES-affirming practices.

Let's Move!

Web site: http://www.letsmove.gov.

In 2010, First Lady Michelle Obama launched the Let's Move! program as part of a goal of eliminating childhood obesity in America within a generation. She enlisted public officials, the food industry, and advocacy groups to raise public awareness about the impact of environmental aspects of obesity. Three of the coordinated aims were to provide healthier foods in schools, ensure that every family has access to healthy, affordable food, and to help and encourage kids to become more physically active. A Let's Move! Web site was created to offer tips and tools on how to raise healthy children at home and in schools. Everyone is encouraged to participate in the President's Challenge to choose from more than 100 activities and exercise (60 minutes per day for children and 30 minutes per day for adults), 5 days a week, for 6 weeks. The site allows exercisers to sign up, log personal activity, compare fitness and physical activity progress with other participants, and even earn a Presidential Active Lifestyle Award.

Mindless Eating

Web site: http://mindlesseating.org/.

This Web site complements Brian Wansink's book *Mindless Eating: Why We Eat More Than We Think*. It has numerous thought-provoking ideas about structuring surroundings to reduce the risk of mindless eating. A "Teaching Toolbox" is a treasure trove of cartoons, Fun in-class activities (K–12 and college), PowerPoint presentations, science fair grants for students (K–12), and understanding and critiquing journal articles.

National Association to Advance Fat Acceptance

Web site: http://www.naafaonline.com/dev2/

Since 1969, the National Association to Advance Fat Acceptance (**NAAFA**), which bills itself as a civil rights organization, has had a mission to promote size acceptance and improve the quality of life for people of any weight or shape. The Web site furnishes information about assessing attitudes, promoting size acceptance, and for healthcare professionals, individuals, employers, and schools. There is a link to "Travel tips for people of size" and the news section reports on NAAFAs ongoing advocacy, public education, and support.

National Center for Complementary and Alternative Medicine

Web site: https://nccih.nih.gov/.

The National Center for Complementary and Integrative Health (NCCIH) is one of the 27 institutes and centers that make up the National Institutes of Health. In December 2014, the agency changed its name from the National Center for Complementary and Alternative Medicine to NCCIH. The term "complementary and alternative medicine" is usually applied when discussing practices and products outside the mainstream of current health systems. The new term "integrative health" emphasizes that incorporating complementary approaches into mainstream health care is becoming more common and desirable. The center supports rigorous scientific methodology to investigate complementary, alternative, and integrative treatments; training researchers; and publishing reliable information for the public and professionals. The Web site includes fact sheets and resources about various types of medical and health strategies. Some of the topics are: "5 Tips: What Consumers Need To Know About Dietary Supplements" and a comprehensive list of "Topics A–Z." There is a link to "Understanding Health News" that describes how to detect the health value of news stories about complementary approaches to health that are often on television, the Internet, and in magazines and newspapers.

Overweight and Obesity

Web site: http://www.cdc.gov/obesity/.

This Centers for Disease Control and Prevention-sponsored gateway provides links to a multitude of Web sites that promote healthy weights for individuals, families, and communities. For example, one link leads to the "Rethink Your Drink" page that shows the calories for a number of drinks and substitutions to help decrease your calories. A 20-ounce bottle of non-diet cola has 227 calories. Try a beverage with zero calories such as diet soda, water, or tea. A 20-ounce medium café latte with whole milk has 265 calories; with fat-free milk it has 125 calories. The section titled "Spread the Word" has links to social media tools and a social marketing Web course. There is a video, "Finding a Balance," with expert perspectives to provide insights into ways caloric or "energy" balance can be achieved and personal stories of how individuals have made changes in their lives to reach this balance. From this site, the user can access hundreds of links to scientific evidence, realistic health tips, brochures, and guides for all aspects of weight management.

Partnership for a Healthier America

Web site: http://www.ahealthieramerica.org/.

The Partnership for a Healthier America (PHA), an independent, nonpartisan organization, was created in 2010, with a mandate to organize the private sector, foundations, media, and local communities to meet the goals of the Let's Move! campaign. The government-private sector collaboration was initiated, based on the concept that industries that shape food availability and physical activity environments should be recognized and included as partners who play an important part in reducing obesity. As one of the first steps when the partnership began, the PHA was committed to bringing healthy, affordable food to millions of people by creating new stores in low-income areas that lacked opportunities to purchase these foods close to home. The PHA has focused on reducing youth obesity and the Web site includes third-party reports on the progress the partners are making. The Web site also has blogs and video messages about PHA activities. There are also quizzes and even songs for a healthy America.

Shape Up America! Cyberkitchen

Web site: http://www.shapeup.org/stmstd/kitchen/page0.php

Shape Up America!, founded in 1994, is a national initiative to promote awareness of obesity as a major public health priority and to provide responsible information on health weight management. The Cyberkitchen is an interactive guide to healthy eating, weight management, and how to balance the food with physical activity. Click on "I'm new here; show me what to do" to tailor "The Kitchen" to individual needs and preferences. Based on age, height, weight, gender, and physical activity, an estimated calorie goal can be adjusted if a goal is to lose or gain weight. There are suggestions as to how to burn extra calories or add extra calories. Daily dietary fat can be monitored using the fat grams calculator. One can choose meals from a selection of breakfasts, lunches, dinners, and snacks. Then, the meals are compared with an individual's calorie goal. Recipes and a shopping list are generated based on the meal choices.

SuperTracker

Web site: https://www.supertracker.usda.gov/.

The U.S. Department of Agriculture-sponsored Super-Tracker is an interactive and personalized tool based on current *Dietary Guidelines for Americans* that allows users to track diet and physical activity, and to compare their diets to MyPlate goals, and their exercise to recommended physical activity guidelines. SuperTracker participants can even receive virtual coaching with tips on what to eat and interesting new exercise ideas. The advice, based on age, weight, sex, and health goals, is customized and one can receive detailed reports of how nutrient intake and lifestyle habits change, or not, over time.

What You Should Know Before You Start a Weight Loss Plan American Academy of Family Physicians

Web site: http://familydoctor.org/familydoctor/en/prevention-wellness/food-nutrition/weight-loss.html.

The American Academy of Family Physicians (AAFP) presents a page on their organization Web site that is dedicated to food and nutrition. Links to "Healthy Food Choices" and "Weight Loss & Diet Plans" display helpful ideas for anyone trying to manage weight. The advice and diet plans are reviewed by physicians and patient education professionals at the AAFP. All the recommendations emphasize that each individual is different and there is no universal diet that will help every person lose weight. Personalized lifestyle changes, including healthful eating and adequate exercise, are the keys to long-term success.

Weight-Control Information Network

Web site: http://www.niddk.nih.gov/health-information/
health-communication-programs/win/Pages/default.aspx.

Weight-Control Information Network (WIN) is an information service of NIDDK at NIH. Its focus is on getting information to the public and media on body weight. WIN covers the range from underweight, normal weight, and obesity. WIN provides information about risks associated with overweight/obesity with special emphasis on diabetes. The WIN Web site is a one-stop site that provides an expansive array of information, tip sheets, fact sheets, and culturally relevant brochures for a range of audiences. From the WIN Health Topics A-Z link, one can view dozens of weight control and healthy living topics listed in alphabetical order. Select a letter to open a link to learn about a disease or condition, diagnostic test, or anatomy topic. Featured topics include: "Choosing a Safe and Successful Weight-loss Program," "Overweight & Obesity Statistics," and "Weight-loss and Nutrition Myths: How Much Do You Really Know?" There is a section specifically for healthcare professionals that has downloadable fact sheets and brochures on weight loss and obesity topics. Links to "Bariatric Surgery for Severe Obesity" and "Medications for the Treatment of Obesity" describe the surgical procedures, types of obesity drugs available, how much weight loss can be expected from these medical interventions, and some of the side effects and risks of the surgeries and medications.

Children and Adolescents Information and Interactive Sites

CDC Growth Charts for Children

Web site: http://www.cdc.gov/growthcharts.

The *CDC Growth Charts* for children are used to compare the growth rates of infants, children, and teens with population norms derived from the data collected in the U.S. National

Health and Nutrition Examination Survey (NHANES), for infants, birth to 36 months, age-related measurements that can be plotted are length, weight, or head circumference. Children and adolescents, 2–20 years, are measured by height and weight for age or BMI for age. BMI ranges for children and teens are also defined so that they take into account normal differences between boys and girls at various ages. The BMI number is plotted on BMI-for-age growth charts specific for either girls or boys to obtain a percentile ranking. The percentile indicates the relative position of the child's BMI number among children of the same sex and age.

Fuel Up to Play 60

Web site: http://www.fueluptoplay60.com/.

Fuel Up to Play 60 is a program founded by the National Dairy Council and National Football League (NFL) in collaboration with USDA that aims to empower students to make healthful choices every day. Students can win prizes, like an NFL player visit or Super Bowl tickets, for eating good-for-you foods, and getting active for at least 60 minutes every day. The site includes fun and focused ways for students to make their school a healthier place. Students can help design and lead these programs or even create their own with help from parents and teachers. Program resources include a wealth of information about nutrition education and physical activity for use in the classroom and at home. The lessons support the 2010 *Dietary Guidelines for Americans*.

Kidnetics

Web site: http:/Kidnetic.com.

Kidnetics is a website for kids and their parents to learn about the body, nutrition, and health in a fun and interactive way. It provides kid-friendly recipes, games, and exciting ways to obtain physical fitness. The International Food Information

Council (IFIC), an organization supported by food, beverage, and agricultural industries, has partnered with America on the Move, Food Marketing Institute, and The President's Council on Physical Fitness and Sports. IFIC partnered with *America on the Move*, *Food Marketing Institute*, and *The President's Council on Physical Fitness and Sports* to create a Web site for kids and their parents to learn about the body, nutrition, and health in a fun and interactive way. IFIC is supported by the food, beverage, and agricultural industries; however, it is listed as a noncommercial site. That means it may not contain advertising or anything for sale.

Media-Smart Youth: Eat, Think, and Be Active

Web site: http://www.nichd.nih.gov/msy/

Created by the Eunice Kennedy Shriver National Institute of Child Health and Human Development, the Media-Smart Youth program is an after-school program designed to help children learn how to make smart food choices. Participants discover how the media can lead to poor health choices in their lives. Educating children about the media is important because many children spend hours watching television, playing video games, or surfing the Web. All these activities take time away from physical activity. They can lead to poor health choices based on the messages they display. This program is available to after-school providers or activity leaders to help children incorporate activities into their daily routines.

MyPlate for Preschoolers

Web site: http://www.choosemyplate.gov/preschoolers.html.

This site encourages healthy eating and physical activity behaviors for children ages 2–5. It includes numerous ideas about daily food plans for picky eaters, sample meal patterns, kitchen activities for kids, and how adults can be a healthy role model for children

MyPlate for Children over Five

Web site: http://www.choosemyplate.gov/children-over-five. html.

This version of MyPlate, geared toward children ages 6–11, bridges the gap between preschoolers and teens. Age-appropriate activities, such as a trip to "Planet Power" are designed to encourage kids to fuel themselves with healthful foods and do physical activity every day. Some tips supplied for parents are how to choose "Kid-friendly vegetables and fruits" and "Cut back on your kid's sweet treats."

We Can! Ways to Enhance Children's Activity & Nutrition

Web site: http://www.nhlbi.nih.gov/health/public/heart/obesity/wecan/

We Can!™ stands for Ways to Enhance Children's Activity & Nutrition. *We Can!* is a national education program designed for parents and caregivers to help children 8–13 years old stay at a healthy weight. The goal of the *We Can!* partnership is to build collaborations around preventive strategies through outreach efforts and leveraging resources and communication channels to disseminate *We Can!* messages and materials to parents, caregivers, and youth ages 8–13 across the United States. Three behaviors are emphasized: improved food choices, increased physical activity, and reduced screen time. The program is summarized by three phrases: Learn it; Live it, Get involved. There are links to science-based educational programs and training opportunities for youth and their parents and families. Each section presents background information and an action plan.

Databases

CDC National Center for Chronic Disease Prevention and Health Promotion, Division of Nutrition, and Physical Activity

Web site: http://www.cdc.gov/nccdphp/dnpao/

This Internet-based, searchable directory presents information on physical activity programs involving state departments of health. It is searchable by state and other key categories, and includes brief program descriptions with information about partner organizations, status scope, target population, setting, purpose, program components, evaluation, and products. Contact information for programs within each state is also provided.

Healthfinder.gov

Web site: www.healthfinder.gov.

This federally sponsored Web site serves as a key resource manager for over 1,400 Web sites about government and non-profit agencies that provide access to the latest and most reliable health information. The Web site is managed by ODPHP under the guidance of expert advisors who are committed to offering quality online health information. Each topic (listed from A to Z) cites the original sources for the content, and every health topic is reviewed and updated at least once a year.

MEDLINEplus® Health Information or US National Library of Medicine and the National Institutes of Health

Web site: http://medlineplus.gov/ or www.nlm.nih.gov/medlineplus.

The National Institutes of Health maintains this Web site with daily updates to present information to health professionals and consumers regarding over 950 diseases and health and wellness issues. The information comes from the National Library of Medicine, the world's largest medical library. There are links that describe the action of prescription drugs, over-the-counter medicines, and nutrition supplements. One can view videos about surgeries, images for diseases or medical treatments, or find out about clinical research trials. The MedlinePlus Web site was created to offer a wide range of free, reliable, and current health information that is accessible anytime and anywhere.

National Center for Health Statistics

Web site: http://www.cdc.gov/nchs.

To provide a broad perspective of the U.S. population's health and influences on health outcomes, the National Center for Health Statistics (NCHS) collects health-related statistics from many other agencies data collection programs. From that data, the NCHS creates interactive data files and also easy-to-understand figures, tables, and reports. For example, data from National Health and Nutrition Examination Survey is used to produce graphics about the prevalence of obesity over time or according to age or ethnicity. The Center draws data from the National Vital Statistics System to display information about birth rates, leading causes of death, and life expectancy. On the attractive and frequently updated Web site, one can get access to facts and figures quickly by following the "FastStats A to Z" link: http://www.cdc.gov/nchs/fastats/.

Nutrition.gov

Web site: http://www.nutrition.gov.

Nutrition.gov is maintained by the staff at the Food and Nutrition Information Center (FNIC) and the National Agricultural Library in cooperation with a panel of food and nutrition expert advisors from agencies within U.S. Department of Agriculture and Department of Health and Human Services. FNIC's staff of trained nutrition professionals, most of whom are registered dietitian nutritionists, provide information on food and human nutrition. This national resource provides access to all online federal government information about nutrition, healthy eating, physical activity, and food safety. There are links to a wide variety of health issues. The site is kept fresh with the latest news and features links to interesting sites.

The online article, "Interested in Losing Weight?" (http://www.nutrition.gov/losingweight) reviews resources and hints such as: "What You Need to Know before Getting Started," "Key Behaviors of Successful Losers," and "Popular Diets." Some of resources are also available in Spanish.

National Nutrient Database

> U.S. Department of Agriculture, Agricultural Research Service
>
> **Web site**: http://ndb.nal.usda.gov/.

The National Nutrient Database, developed and maintained by the national Nutrient Data Laboratory, provides details of nutrient content for over 8,000 foods. This information can be used by consumers to assess their diets, by government agencies to set nutrition standards, and by food companies to describe and evaluate commercial food products.

National Weight Control Registry

> **Web site**: http://www.nwcr.ws.

The National Weight Control Registry (NWCR) is a project developed in 1994 by Dr. Rena Wing and Dr. James Hill to help identify those individuals who have succeeded at long-term weight maintenance and to examine the strategies that were successful. Participants may register if they have maintained at least a 30-pound weight loss for more than a year. With more than 5,000 people participating in the NWCR, the researchers found that the average weight loss for all enrollees is 66 pounds. Follow-up questionnaires indicate that most weight is kept off for more than five years, and weight loss is maintained by a variety of personally designed diet and exercise strategies. To continue to be successful at managing weight, 98 percent of participants say they modify their food intake in some way and 90 percent have increased their physical activity to about 1 hour per day. The Web site provides information about how to join the Registry, research study results, and success stories from participants.

Nutrition Data: Know What You Eat

> **Web site**: http://nutritiondata.self.com/

Since its launch in 2003, the *Nutrition Data* Web site has aimed to provide a comprehensive nutrition analysis database that is free, accessible, and understandable to all. Based on the amounts of nutrients in foods listed on the USDA's National Nutrient Database for Standard Reference, this database also includes the latest nutrition information from restaurants and the food industry. Opportunities to interact with the Nutrition Data tools include the ability to enter personal recipes to be analyzed and to print standard format Nutrition Facts Labels for any combination of foods. A "My Tracking" tool provides a way to assess daily calorie consumption and to evaluate intake of more than 130 nutrients. The "BMI & Calories Burned Calculator" provides an estimate of the calories burned by various types of exercise for a given BMI. The "Nutrition Data's Better Choices Diet"™ is a diet plan that includes tips to reduce caloric intake without increasing hunger.

WHO Global InfoBase

Web site: http://www.who.int/bmi/index.jsp.

The Global Infobase on Body Mass Index is an interactive tool where readers can view the prevalence of adult weight categories (underweight, overweight, and obesity) in countries throughout the world. The World Health Organization maintains and regularly updates the database and presents the information as graphs, maps, data tables, and documents. Each of these may be manipulated by clicking on the respective tabs so data can be displayed by country or year. On this Web site, one can compare and contrast the rates and trends of obesity in any country to get an estimate of worldwide extent of the obesity problem.

Calculators and Counters

BMI Calculators

BMI is a number based on height and weight of an individual that may be determined using an online calculator or table or by using either of the following equations:

BMI = weight (lb)/[height (in)] 2 × 703 (standard units of measure)

BMI = weight (kg)/[height (m)]2 (metric units of measure) (kg = kilogram, m = meter, lb = pound, and in = inch).

Adult BMI Calculator

Centers for Disease Control and Prevention

Web site: http://www.cdc.gov/healthyweight/assessing/bmi/ adult_bmi/english_bmi_calculator/bmi_calculator.html.

By entering height and weight, adults—individuals 20 years and older—may use this calculator to determine their BMI and weight category (underweight, normal weight, overweight, and obese).

BMI Calculator for Children and Teens

Centers for Disease Control and Prevention
Web site: http://nccd.cdc.gov/dnpabmi/Calculator.aspx.

The "BMI Calculator for Children and Teens" is designed to calculate the BMI specifically for young people aged 2–19 years old. In addition to height and weight, age, and sex are also entered into the calculation to provide a BMI-for-age estimate.

Body Mass Index Table

National Heart, Lung, and Blood Institute

Web site: http:www.nhlbi.nih.gov/guidelines/obesity/bmi_ tbl.htm.

One can determine BMI by looking at the intersection of an individual's height and body weight in this table. There is a pdf version for printing.

The Calorie Counter 4th Edition

Annette B. Natow, Ph.D., Jo-Ann Heslin, M.A., R.D.

Pocket Books, a division of Simon & Schuster Inc., 2007. 688pp.

ISBN: 1416509828

The calorie counter provides information, such as calories, fat, protein, carbohydrates, and other nutrients, for items at chain restaurants, brand name foods found in grocery stores, energy bars and drinks, and ethnic foods. This book is easy to carry in the pocket or purse while shopping or dining out. There are over 20,000 listings.

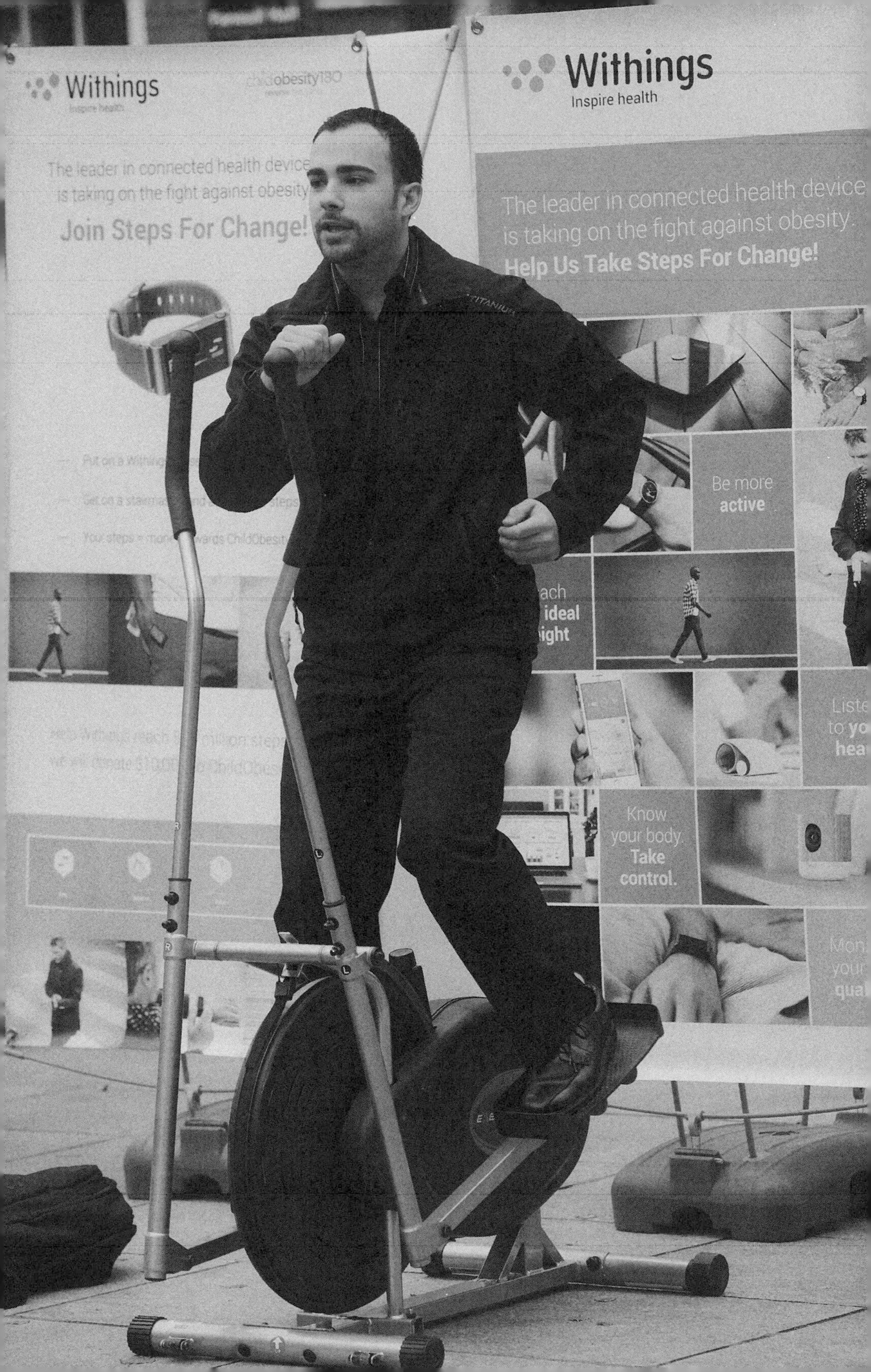
Withings
Inspire health
Join Steps For Change!
Withings
Inspire health
The leader in connected health device
is taking on the fight against obesity.
Help Us Take Steps For Change!
Be more
active
Know
your body.
Take
control.

The issue of obesity is not a consequence of any single factor. The condition does not exist in a vacuum. It is the result of interactions among genetics, physiology, behavior, and even politics and economics. This chapter presents a chronology of important events occurring from 1942 to 2015 that demonstrate how individual, government, scientific, and corporate attitudes and opinions have changed during that time. The timeline allows the reader to recognize how nutrition, activity, behavioral, pharmaceutical, and surgical approaches to obesity management have changed. Year by year, one can see an increasing role for the federal government as agencies and programs are formed and assessed. This decades-long look at many factors that contribute to obesity and at the people and programs attempting to prevent and treat obesity may be a useful guide toward more effective obesity management in the future.

1942   Louis Dublin, a statistician at Metropolitan Life Insurance Company (MLIC), grouped about four million people who were insured with Metropolitan Live into categories based on their height, body frame (small, medium, or large), and weight. People who maintained their body weights at the

---

A man uses exercise equipment to benefit charity at the Obesity Week 2014 conference in Boston, Massachusetts. It is now generally accepted that it is necessary to combine exercise with a healthy diet to combat obesity and the health risks that accompany it. Over the past decades, attitudes and opinions about which are the most important obesity management components—nutrition, activity, behavioral, and/or medical approaches—have continued to evolve. (Aynsley Floyd/AP Images for Withings)

average for 25-year olds lived the longest. As insurance companies look for criteria by which to judge the desirability of applicants, these became the acceptable height-weight ranges for men and women and are called "ideal weights."

1943   In 1943, enough of the U.S. population is above the ideal body weight (IBW) that the MLIC declares, "Overweight is so common that it constitutes a national health problem of the first order."

1951   Tillie Lewis starts a new food company (based in Stockton, California) that offers new low-calorie products. Lewis becomes one of the earliest marketers of diet foods with her Tasti-Diet line of artificially sweetened fruits, soft drinks, puddings, jellies, and chocolate sauce.

1952   Dr. Lester Breslow popularizes the idea of optimum weight for health. In a classic paper Breslow, notes that "One out of six well people . . . are 20 percent or more overweight" and that "Weight control is a major public health problem."

1954   The first bariatric surgery to be submitted to a peer-reviewed journal is performed. Drs. Arnold Kremen and John Linner at the University of Minnesota are studying nutrition absorption in dogs. They discover that the dogs lose weight after they undergo operations that bypass much of their intestines. In Dr. Linner's private surgical practice, one of his patients asks him to use the technique on her in the hopes that she, too, will lose weight. With the successful results of that procedure, bariatric surgery is born.

1956   President Dwight Eisenhower establishes the *President's Council on Physical Fitness and Sports* out of concern that Americans are becoming less active. The program is a partnership between the public, private, and nonprofit sectors of society. The spark to develop The Council comes from John Kelly, who was better known as the father of the actress Grace Kelly. John Kelly was a wartime physical fitness officer who believes that the current affluent lifestyle makes life so easy and effortless that adults and children are rapidly losing muscle tone.

1956   Jack LaLanne brings his fitness and diet television program into living rooms throughout the United States. His popular television series, "The Jack LaLanne Show," encourages viewers to get up from the chair and work out. Jack's belief that daily, vigorous, systematic exercise and proper diet are keys to good health is an idea that is accepted and supported by medical professionals in future years.

1959   The MLIC replaces the term "ideal weight" with "desirable weight," when it is discovered that these weights are associated with the lowest mortality among people from the United States and Canada who purchased life insurance policies from 1935 to 1954.

1960   Metrecal, a diet drink in a can, is introduced by the Mead Johnson Company as a weight loss aid. Metrecal is a complete low-calorie meal that does not require calorie counting or food preparation. It is the first in a long line of commercial liquid diets that will include products such as SlimFast beverages.

1963   Jean Neiditch, a housewife from Queens, New York, starts the Weight Watchers Club basing it on a plan that helped her lose more than 50 pounds. Each week, she invites her friends to her home to discuss how to lose weight. The Club is successful, as it provides motivation, mutual support, and encouragement from people who are all working on weight loss or maintenance. Members can become meeting leaders and share the story of their personal success with others. This enterprise will grow into Weight Watchers International, a successful business with about a million members worldwide attending 400,000 groups each week.

1964   Dr. G. J. Hamwi develops a simple way to estimate ideal body weight (IBW). His formulas for IBW will be a popular method used in clinical practice for decades to come.

1967   Surgeon Edward E. Mason at the University of Iowa is called the "father of gastric bypass surgery" for weight loss. Previous to this version, surgeons would just remove part of the intestine, a procedure called gastrointestinal bypass, to reduce the number of calories the body could absorb. For a further reduction in food intake, Dr. Mason used staples to create a small pouch in the top of the stomach. Patients would feel full eating less since there was not much room for food.

1970   Jaw wiring is used for weight loss. This orthodontic procedure prevents the mouth from opening more than a few centimeters. As a form of weight control it prevents consumption of solid food, thus causing a reduction in calorie intake. It is suggested as a method to be tried before surgery is attempted.

1970   Obesity is estimated to exist in 4 percent of children and 13 percent of adults in the United States.

1972   *Dr. Atkins' Diet Revolution* is published. Dr. Robert Atkins recommends eating a diet high in protein and fat and low in carbohydrates. He believes that by reducing carbohydrates, the body will burn excess fat for fuel, and he uses the plan to resolve his own overweight condition. Although the book is a bestseller, the Atkins diet is considered outside of the medical mainstream for the next 30 years.

1974   The first International Congress on Obesity is held in London, Great Britain. There are 500 attendees from 30 countries. This meeting is organized in recognition of the fact that there is a need for continuing international assemblies of obesity experts and policy makers.

1980   Body mass index (BMI) becomes an international standard for obesity measurement.

1980   Liposuction is introduced in the United States. With the introduction of liposuction, the removal of localized fatty deposits and body contouring becomes the most requested and fastest growing cosmetic surgery procedure.

1982   The first nonprofit professional organization to study obesity is established. The North American Association for the Study of Obesity, which later became The Obesity Society (TOS), is committed to encouraging research on the causes and treatment of obesity, and to keeping the medical community and public informed of new advances.

1983   The MLIC tables are revised again, when it is discovered that some heavier people live longer than lower weight individuals. According to height, the new tables increase the desirable weight 2–13 pounds for men and 3–8 pounds for women.

1984   Dr. Michael Weintraub's research on obese patients shows that a combination of two drugs, phentermine and fenfluramine, are more effective at producing weight loss than either of the drugs alone, and in lower dosages with fewer side effects. Fenfluramine has been used for decades as a Food and Drug Administration (FDA)-approved weight loss medication, but the combination is not yet sanctioned by the FDA.

1985   The National Institutes of Health (NIH) classifies obesity as a disease. Formerly, obesity was thought to result from the single adverse behavior of eating inappropriate quantities. Studies that show specific biochemical alterations occur in humans and experimental animals in response to environmental food and activity factors indicate that obesity meets the definition of a disease.

1985–1998   BMI risk categories for Americans are defined. Definition of overweight in U.S. government publications is a BMI of at least 27.3 for women and 27.8 for men.

1988   The 7-Eleven fast-food outlets introduce the giant 64-ounce Double Gulp® beverage—one of the biggest fountain soft drinks on the market—containing nearly 800 calories.

1989   A research study by Thomas Wadden and others shows that 98 percent of dieters regain all lost weight within five years.

1990   During this decade, leptin is discovered by several groups in obese mice that carry a gene that makes them unable to produce any leptin. The hormone regulates energy expenditure and food intake in rodents. While there can be thousands of leptin-deficient mice, fewer than 10 people in the entire world are obese because of absolute leptin deficiency.

1990   The Nutrition Labeling and Education Act (NLEA) is signed into law. This act is a new mandate for food manufacturers to provide a label with nutrient and calorie content for their products.

1991   An NIH panel endorses gastric bypass surgery for obesity. The NIH experts conclude that surgical alterations of the digestive system are an effective option for severely obese people who have not been successful with more moderate weight-reduction strategies.

1991   The National Heart, Lung, and Blood Institute (NHLBI) establishes the Obesity Education Initiative (OEI) with the aim of decreasing cardiovascular disease (CVD) and type 2 diabetes, by reducing the prevalence of overweight and increasing physical activity in Americans.

1992   *Dr. Atkins' New Diet Revolution* is published. This updated version of Dr. Atkins' diet becomes very popular and his company, Atkins Nutritionals, will eventually have revenues that reach $100 million a year.

1992   The diet drug Fen-Phen (fenfluramin and phentermine) is marketed aggressively as a magic weight loss pill. Hundreds of clinics open specifically to prescribe this weight loss medication. There is mass marketing of this new drug combination and the number of prescriptions written for Fen-Phen grows from 60,000 in 1992 to 18 million in 1996.

1993   The National Weight Control Registry (NWCR) is founded at the University of Colorado by Dr. James Hill and Dr. Rena Wing. The NWCR is a long-term study of individuals 18 years and older, who have successfully maintained at least a 30-pound weight loss for a year or more.

1993   In the first decision of its kind, a Federal court of appeals panel rules that job discrimination against severely obese people violates Federal disabilities law.

1995   The International Obesity Task Force (IOTF) is established by Dr. W. P. T. James. A major concern of IOTF is reversing the increase in childhood obesity around the world.

1995   The World Health Organization (WHO) recommends a classification for three grades of overweight using BMI cutoff points of 25, 30, and 40. The IOTF suggests an additional cutoff point of 35.

1996   FDA approves the noncaloric fat substitute olestra for use in chips and crackers. The first snack foods made with Olean are introduced in Iowa, Wisconsin, and Colorado by Frito-Lay. The foods are so popular that a store in Cedar Rapids takes mail orders from snack lovers all across the country.

1997   A Fen-Phen link to heart valve damage is established when the Mayo Clinic reports 24 cases of heart valve disease in people who use the diet medication. In September 1997, with growing evidence linking the drugs to potentially fatal heart and lung disorders, manufacturer American Home Products removes the drug from the market.

1997   In November 1997, a few months after the withdrawal of Fen-Phen, the FDA approves Meridia, a drug that falls into the same class of many antidepressants such as Prozac. It is marketed as an alternative to Fen-Phen.

1997   The FDA approves orlistat (brand name Xenical) as a prescription medication to help people lose weight and Hoffmann-La Roche Inc. releases it onto the market. Orlistat is a lipase inhibitor that acts in the gastrointestinal tract to block the absorption of fat by inhibiting pancreatic enzymes. Unlike other diet drugs, it does not interfere with brain chemistry.

1998   An expert panel convened by NIH releases a report that defines overweight as a BMI between 25 and 29.9, and obesity as a BMI of 30 or greater. These definitions will become widely used by the federal government and the broader medical and scientific communities. The cut points are based on evidence that health risks increase more steeply in individuals with a BMI greater than 25.

1998   The *NHLBI Clinical Guidelines on the Identification, Evaluation, and Treatment of Overweight and Obesity in Adults* is published and distributed to primary care physicians and other health care professionals, so they can begin using the new guidelines to treat obese patients. The report lays out a new approach for assessing overweight and obesity, and it establishes evidence-based principles for safe and effective weight loss for the first time. The guidelines also provide practical strategies for implementing the recommendations.

1999 Studies show leptin is not effective for human weight loss. The discovery of the fat-regulating hormone, leptin created great excitement when it was believed that injecting obese patients with leptin could produce easy weight loss. The hope among scientists and obese people is dashed when clinical trials in humans conducted in 1999 show that the hormone is not effective, as only a small amount of weight was lost even with high doses of leptin.

1999 Singer Carnie Wilson has gastric bypass surgery and allows the actual procedure to be broadcast live over the Internet. The broadcast is viewed by more than 500,000 people. The 31-year-old weighed more than 300 pounds before the procedure that reduced her stomach to the size of an egg.

1999 Each American consumes an average of 155 pounds of caloric sweeteners (sugars, honey, corn syrups) that amount to more than 50 teaspoonfuls of added sugars per person per day.

2000 An historical moment occurs when the estimated number of overweight people in the world exceeds those who are underweight.

2000 Jared Fogle loses 425 pounds eating low-fat sandwiches from the Subway food outlet. The 22-year-old, 6 foot 2 inch, Indiana University college student says he created a 1,000 calorie-a-day Subway diet consisting of not much more than Subway sandwiches for a year. Jared proves that a low-fat, calorie-conscious, convenient diet can work.

2000 In January 2000, the U.S. Department of Health and Human Services (HHS) launches *Healthy People 2010*, a comprehensive, nationwide health promotion and disease prevention agenda. Each objective has a target to be achieved by the year 2010. Targets that are directly related to obesity are to: increase the proportion of adults who are at a healthy weight to 60 percent of Americans; reduce the proportion of adults who are obese to 15 percent or less of the population; reduce the proportion of children and adolescents who are overweight or obese to 5 percent of the population.

2000   The IOTF Childhood Obesity Working Group publishes standard definitions for overweight and obesity in childhood. Up until this point, there has been a lack of agreement about the definition of overweight and obesity in childhood and adolescence.

2001   In the 2001 *Surgeon General's Call to Action to Prevent and Decrease Overweight and Obesity*, U.S. Surgeon General David Satcher declares that obesity is a public health epidemic that could be the cause of as much preventable disease and death as cigarette smoking. He releases a call to action to promote the recognition of obesity as a health problem and to develop programs to treat obesity and encourage people to change their eating and exercise habits.

2002   The Federal Trade Commission (FTC) releases a report titled *Weight Loss Advertising: An Analysis of Current Trends*, indicating that the use of false and misleading claims in weight loss advertising is widespread with more than half of weight loss ads making claims that are misleading, lack proof, or are obviously false. The FTC warns that some weight loss supplements lack safety warnings and can be dangerous.

2002   Obesity treatment gets a boost when the Internal Revenue Service (IRS) recognizes obesity as a disease and allows medical tax deductions for medically valid obesity treatments.

2003   The FTC launches a campaign to educate U.S. media professionals about false weight loss claims. The promotion, called the *Red Flag Campaign*, is an attempt to expose advertisements that are fraudulent and scientifically impossible. The FTC produces a reference guide so that media outlets can screen out bogus claims by checking through the list without having to go into in-depth investigations on their own.

2003   At a congressional briefing in 2003, Surgeon General Richard H. Carmona declares that obesity is an epidemic and he speaks about the "Obesity Crisis in America". He calls obesity a health crisis that is the fastest growing cause of disease and death in America.

2003   In the first ever policy statement exclusively focused on identifying and preventing childhood obesity, the American Academy of Pediatrics asks pediatricians to go beyond their routine tracking of height and weight. The group wants doctors to use the body mass index for children and adolescents. The policy instructs pediatricians to promote healthy eating and physical activity at each office visit.

2003   In the United States, young people spend an average of almost 6.5 hours a day with electronic media such as televisions radios, video players and computers. That is an increase of more than an hour since 2000.

2004   The population obesity rate for American children, ages 6–11 years, is 19 percent, and for 12–19-year-old adolescents, the rate is 17 percent. Foretelling a future with more obese children and adolescents, data this year shows that more than 10 percent of younger children (ages 2–5) are overweight. That is up from 7 percent in 1994.

2004   The *Strategic Plan for NIH Obesity Research* is released. The NIH Research Task Force publishes a multifaceted agenda for the study of behavioral and environmental causes of obesity, along with the study of genetic and biologic causes. The Plan details coordination of obesity research across NIH.

2004   In February of this year, the FDA bans the sale of all dietary supplements in the United States that contain ephedrine. The agency says they create an unreasonable risk of illness and injury.

2004   A controversial independent film called *Supersize Me* by Martin Spurlock is introduced as an exploration of the prevalence of obesity in the United States. Spurlock eats only food from the McDonald's menu for a month. He starts as a healthy man and becomes overweight and experiences issues with his health.

2004   Research study reveals that 30 percent of children eat fast food on a daily basis. The findings suggest that fast-food consumption has increased fivefold among children since 1970.

2004   To promote healthy lifestyles for adults and children in all countries, WHO develops the *Global Strategy on Diet, Physical Activity and Health* (DPAS). This is endorsed by the 57th World Health Assembly in May 2004.

2004   The IOTF report, *Obesity in children and young people: A crisis in public health*, sends an alert that childhood obesity is increasing in both developed and developing countries. The report warns that obesity significantly increases the risk that children may develop type 2 diabetes, heart disease, and a variety of adverse health consequences which may not become evident until adulthood.

2004   McDonald's fast-food outlets plan to phase out Super Size french fries and soft drinks as the world's largest restaurant chain promotes its "Eat Smart, Be Active" initiative. McDonald's is adding salads and moving to provide more fruit, vegetable, and yogurt options with children's Happy Meals. The new program is designed to put McDonald's in a position of being part of the solution to the obesity issue, rather than part of the problem.

2005   The *2005 Dietary Guidelines for Americans* are released. Each 5-year revision of the guidelines is based on analysis of the latest scientific information by the Dietary Guidelines Advisory Committee and forms the basis for government program and policy development. So, individuals can follow the guidelines in their daily lives, the dietary recommendations are presented as healthy eating patterns such as the U.S. Department of Agriculture (USDA) Food Guide and the DASH (Dietary Approaches to Stop Hypertension) Eating Plan. The guidelines are depicted graphically as a Food Guide Pyramid (FGP) that recommends types and amounts of foods from seven food groups and daily physical activity.

2005   On April 14, a judge in the Federal district court overturns the FDA ephedra ban as a result of a suit brought by the Nutraceutical Corporation, a supplement manufacturer. The judge concludes that there is not enough scientific evidence to prove that those products with 10 milligrams or less of ephedrine in a daily dose posed a health risk.

2005   A team of experts on the Social Security Advisory Board concludes that the steady rise in human life expectancy during the past two centuries may soon come to an end. The epidemic of obesity and related health risks could cause decline in Americans' life expectancy and could cancel out the life-extending benefits of advances in medicine, and that young people, who are becoming obese at unprecedented rates, will experience the greatest loss of longevity. This prediction leads to the controversial idea that children today may live less healthy and shorter lives than their parents.

2005   A study reports that 46 percent of U.S. women and 33 percent of U.S. men said they were trying to lose weight.

2006   A federal appeals court reinstates the FDA ban on ephedra-containing supplements. The court rules that more than 19,000 adverse events reported to the FDA are enough to uphold the initial ban. The FDA declares that no dose of ephedrine in dietary supplements is safe and that sale of these products is illegal.

2006   In this year, the southeastern region of the United States has the highest prevalence of obesity and overweight. With prevalence equal to or greater than 30 percent of their population, Mississippi and West Virginia lead all the states in the number of citizens who are obese.

2008   New York City's Board of Health becomes the first agency to require that any restaurant chain with 15 or more nationwide outlets show calorie information on menus, menu boards, and food tags. Advocates say this paves the way for other local and state governments to pass similar menu labeling measures.

2006 The Robert Wood Johnson Foundation requests that IOM have an expert committee examine the progress that had been made in preventing childhood obesity in the United States. The resulting report, *Progress in Preventing Childhood Obesity: How Do We Measure Up?* presents specific actions for childhood obesity prevention. Lack of a system for monitoring progress was identified as a stumbling block to evaluating on-going programs. The committee encouraged continuing surveillance and assessment systems to track effectiveness of existing nutrition programs.

2007 An over-the-counter version of the prescription weight loss drug, orlistat, is approved by the U.S. Food and Drug Administration. This is the first time that the FDA has found that an over-the-counter weight loss product actually works. The drug, sold under the brand name Alli, is a reduced strength version of Xenical and works in the same way as it decreases absorption of fat in the intestines. In addition to using the drug, Alli purchasers are encouraged to follow an online diet plan that includes menus and shopping lists and to join a network of other Alli users who provide support.

2007 The American Medical Association (AMA) begins a campaign to educate physicians about how to prevent and manage childhood obesity. The goal is to introduce obesity training as part of undergraduate, graduate, and continuing medical education programs. The committee creates 22 recommendations for health care professionals who provide obesity care to apply in their practices.

2007 Progress toward coordinating the work of the federal and state government's existing childhood obesity prevention programs was made when the HHS created the Childhood Overweight and Obesity Prevention Initiative. The Initiative encourages community-based interventions, such as the NIH We Can! (Ways to Enhance Children's Activity and Nutrition) program, the President's Council on Physical Fitness and Sports' National Fitness Challenge and the National Center for Physical Development and Outdoor Play, which will help improve outdoor play for children in Head Start programs.

2007   The National Center on Health Statistics report, *Obesity Among Adults in the United States—No Change Since 2003–2004*, is the latest analysis based on the National Health and Nutrition Examination Survey data. This may be the first sign that the obesity epidemic could be peaking as a result of prevention and management programs sponsored by the government and healthcare organizations and by individuals' personal effort to control weight. While the obesity prevalence at this time point has not measurably increased in the past few years, levels are still high. More than one-third of adults (over 72 million people) were obese in 2005–2006. This includes 33.3 percent of men and 35.3 percent of women. These percentages are not statistically different from 2003–2004, when 31.1 percent of men were obese and 33.2 percent of women were obese.

2008   At 97 years old, Jack LaLanne, known as the Godfather of the American fitness movement, is inducted into the California Hall of Fame by California First Lady Maria Shriver.

2008   In collaboration with the Robert Wood Johnson Foundation, the IOM establishes the *Standing Committee on Childhood Obesity Prevention*. This committee will aid in integrating ideas and programs from government, academia, and corporate sectors, and will report on the most promising solutions to the prevention of childhood obesity. It will continue to monitor progress toward implementing the recommendations of its first report on Preventing Childhood Obesity.

2010   The federal Affordable Care Act (ACA) is established and it expands benefits and coverage of services for obesity prevention. It also includes a section on nutrition labeling requirements. The ACA requires chain restaurants with 20 or more locations to post calorie and nutrition information on menus, menu boards, drive through displays, and certain vending machines.

2010   First Lady Michelle Obama launches the Let's Move! Program, which has the ambitious goal of eliminating childhood obesity within a generation. The First Lady aims to raise public awareness about the environmental aspects of obesity as the initiative brings together public officials, the food industry, and advocacy groups to find solutions.

2010   The Task Force on Childhood Obesity is formed as a complement to the Let's Move! initiative to develop a coordinated strategy, identify key benchmarks, and outline a national action plan for addressing the problems of childhood obesity.

2010   The HHS unveils *Healthy People 2020*, the nation's new 10-year goals and objectives for health promotion and disease prevention. The agency also launches a newly redesigned Healthy People Web site and Healthy People eLearning, an online educational resource designed to help students and health professionals learn how to reach the Nation's health goals.

2011   An updated *Strategic Plan for NIH Obesity Research* enlarges the previous themes and encourages further investigations into the fresh opportunities presented by technology advances, which emerged in the years since the publication of NIH's first strategic plan in 2004.

2011   The new *2010 Dietary Guidelines for Americans*, which emphasize balancing calories with physical activity to manage weight, are issued in January.

2011   MyPlate replaces USDA food guide pyramid. Now, dietary guidelines are graphically displayed as portions of food on a plate.

2012   Two drugs for weight management Qsymia (phentermine and topiramate) and Belviq (lorcaserin) are approved by the FDA. They are the first drugs to be approved in over a decade since orlistat was allowed in 1997.

2012   The *Healthy People 2010 Final Review* presents a quantitative end-of-decade assessment of progress in achieving the Healthy People 2010 objectives and goals. The result is that no progress was made toward the Healthy People 2010 target of 15 percent reduction in obesity in the United States. Instead, prevalence of obesity increased 47.8 percent. The proportion of adults in the population who were obese rose from 23 to 34 percent. During the same period, obesity increased in children, from 11 to 17 percent and in adolescents from 11 to 18 percent, moving away from the 2010 targets of just 5 percent. The conclusions that can be drawn from this 2008 report is that Americans have made little progress toward the HP 2010 targets.

2013   The Healthy Weight Commitment Foundation, a group of 16 leading food and beverage companies, cuts 6.4 trillion calories from products sold to American consumers, exceeding its pledge by more than 600 percent. In 2007, the companies had vowed to remove 1 trillion calories from the marketplace by 2012.

2013   An update to the 1998 NHLBI *Clinical Guidelines on the Identification, Evaluation, and Treatment of Overweight and Obesity in Adults* is published. The 2013 *Guidelines* are based on up-to-date scientific evidence reviews. A set of treatment recommendations is also developed to help primary care providers, since most clinicians receive no current training in management of obesity.

2013   The American Medical Association officially approves a policy that recognizes obesity as a disease that deserves medical attention and insurance coverage as do other diseases. As a respected representative of American medicine, the AMA opinion can influence policy makers to do more to support interventions and research to prevent and treat obesity. The recognition could induce physicians to pay more attention to the condition and spur more insurers to pay for obesity treatment and prevention.

2014   The Office of Personnel Management, which oversees federal employee health benefits, announces that federal insurance plans may not deny coverage of FDA-approved weight loss medications. The announcement notes that obesity cannot be considered simply a lifestyle condition or that weight loss treatment is only cosmetic. This move by the U.S. government may lead commercial insurance providers to also cover weight loss medications in their plans.

2014   The FDA approves Contrave, the third new prescription weight loss pill since 2012, which combines two medications already on the market: bupropion an antidepressant and naltrexone an anti-addiction drug. It's also approved for those not obese but overweight with risk factors such as high blood pressure, high cholesterol, or diabetes.

2015   *Healthy People 2020 Leading Health Indicators: Progress Update* describes the headway toward meeting selected Leading Health Indicators (LHI). The LHI, a subset of Healthy People objectives, assess high-priority health issues. The obesity-related LHIs show that there has been a dramatic increase in obesity in the United States and, although there has been some leveling off in recent years, rates remain at historically high levels. Between 2005 and 2008 and between 2009 and 2012, the obesity rate among adults aged 20 and older increased about 4 percent, from 33.9 percent to 35.3 percent, moving away from the Healthy People 2020 target of 30.5 percent. Between 2005 and 2008 and between 2009 and 2012, the obesity rate among children and adolescents aged 2–19 increased about 5 percent, from 16.1 percent to 16.9 percent, moving away from the Healthy People 2020 target of 14.5 percent. Similar to the evaluation of the 2010 targets, Americans still are not making progress toward the Healthy People targets.

2015   Burger King drops soft drinks from its children's meal menu. This was the latest change at a fast-food chain as advocacy groups urge restaurants to promote healthier eating for children. Burger King followed the lead of McDonald's, which dropped soft drinks from the Happy Meal menu list in 2013, and Wendy's, which made a similar change in late 2014.

2015   HHS and USDA jointly release and publish the eighth edition of *Dietary Guidelines for Americans*. The report is based on input from the public and recommendations of the Dietary Guidelines Advisory Committee (DGAC). The DGAC examined the *Dietary Guidelines for Americans*, 2010, to determine topics for which new scientific evidence was available that could be applied to the 2015 edition of the *Guidelines*. The DGAC's work was guided by the reality that about two-thirds of U.S. adults are overweight or obese. So, the 2015 *Guidelines* focuses on foods and beverages that help achieve and maintain a healthy weight, promote health, and prevent disease.

Glossary

Adipocytes: Fat cells.

Adipose tissue: Fat tissue in the body.

Anorexiant: A drug, process, or event that leads to anorexia or lack of appetite.

Appetite: Feelings of hunger and desire to eat.

Bariatric: Pertaining to bariatrics, the field of medicine concerned with obesity and weight loss.

Bariatric surgery: Also known as gastrointestinal surgery, it is surgery on the stomach and/or intestines to help patients with extreme obesity to lose weight.

BIA: Bioelectrical impedance analysis is a way to estimate the amount of body weight that is fat and nonfat by measuring the speed of a low-level electrical current as it moves through the body.

Blood glucose: Glucose in the blood stream; blood sugar.

BMI: Body Mass Index relates an individual's weight relative to their height. BMI is a person's weight in kilograms (kg) divided by their height in meters (m) squared. It also can be calculated by multiplying weight in pounds by 703, and then dividing that number by the individual's height in inches squared. The easiest way to figure BMI is to look it up in a table.

Calipers: A metal or plastic tool similar to a compass used to measure the diameter of an object. The skinfold thickness in several parts of the body can be measured with skin calipers to determine the lean body mass.

Calorie: A unit of energy in food. Calories in foods may come from carbohydrates, proteins, fats, and alcohol. Carbohydrates and proteins have 4 calories per gram. Fat has 9 calories per gram. Alcohol has 7 calories per gram.

Carbohydrate: There are two kinds of carbohydrates—simple carbohydrates and complex carbohydrates; simple carbohydrates are sugars and complex carbohydrates include both starches and fiber. Carbohydrates have 4 calories per gram. They are found naturally in foods such as breads, pasta, cereals, fruits, vegetables, and milk and dairy products.

Central fat distribution or abdominal fat: Waist circumference is an index of body fat distribution. In android type (apple shaped) patterns, fat is deposited around the waist and upper abdominal area, and appears most often in men. The gynoid type (pear shaped) distribution of body fat is usually seen in women. The fat is deposited around the hips, thighs, and buttocks.

Childhood (pediatric) obesity: Though the term "childhood obesity" is commonly used, most healthcare providers refrain from using the term "obesity" in relation to children and adolescents. Instead, the condition is referred to as "overweight."

Childhood overweight: Children are classified as "overweight" if their weight ranks above the 95th percentile for age. This class represents the most severe weight classification for children and corresponds to a BMI (body mass index) of at least 30—the same indicator used to classify adult obesity.

Comorbidities: Two or more diseases or conditions existing together in an individual.

CVD: Cardiovascular disease is a disease of the heart or blood vessels; any abnormal condition characterized by dysfunction of the heart or blood vessels.

DEXA: Dual energy X-ray absortiometry is a method used to estimate total body fat and percent of body fat.

Dexfenfluramine: A weight loss drug, in a class of drugs called anorectics which decrease appetite. This drug, sold in the

United States under the brand name Redux, was withdrawn from the U.S. market in 1997 because of its association with heart valve dysfunction.

Diabetes: Any of several metabolic disorders marked by increased blood glucose, excessive discharge of urine, and persistent thirst.

Diastolic blood pressure: The minimum pressure that remains within the artery when the heart is at rest.

Diet: What a person eats and drinks or any type of eating plan.

Energy balance: The state in which the total energy intake equals total energy needs.

Energy deficit: A state in which total energy intake is less than total energy needed.

Energy expenditure: The amount of energy measured in calories that a person uses to breathe, circulate blood, digest food, maintain posture, and to be physically active.

Ephedrine: A sympathomimetic drug that can be appetite suppressant. It stimulates thermogenesis, or the generation of body heat.

Epidemic: The occurrence of more cases of a disease than would be expected in a community or region during a given time period. From the Greek epi-, upon + demos, people or population = epidemos.

Fat: A major source of energy in the diet. All food fats have nine calories per gram. Fat stores in the body are called adipose tissue.

Fenfluramine: A weight loss drug, in a class of drugs called anorectics which decrease appetite. This drug is sold in the United States under the brand name Pondimin. It was withdrawn from the U.S. market in 1997 because of its association with heart valve dysfunction.

Gastric banding: An obesity surgery option that limits the amount of food the stomach can hold by sectioning it off with a band near its upper end. The band creates a small pouch, which delays the emptying of food from the pouch and causes a feeling of fullness.

Gastric bypass: A surgical procedure that combines the creation of small stomach pouch to restrict food intake with the construction of a bypass of the duodenum to prevent food absorption of some food.

Genotype: Describes the entire genetic makeup of an individual or the hereditary factors that define fundamental constitution of an organism.

Glucose: A building block for most carbohydrates. Digestion causes some carbohydrates to break down into glucose. After digestion, glucose is carried in the blood and goes to body cells where it is used for energy or is stored.

High blood pressure: Another word for hypertension. An optimal blood pressure is less than 120/80 millimeter of mercury (mmHg). With high blood pressure, the heart works harder and chances of a stroke, heart attack, and kidney problems are greater.

Hypertension: Abnormally elevated blood pressure.

Incidence: The rate at which a certain event occurs (i.e., in epidemiology, it is the number of new cases of a specific disease occurring during a certain period).

Insulin: A hormone made by the pancreas [see definition] that helps move glucose (sugar) from the blood to muscles and other tissues. Insulin controls blood sugar levels.

LBI: Lean body mass is the weight of the body minus the fat mass.

LCD: A low-calorie diet is a caloric restriction of about 800–1,500 calories (approximately 12–15 kcal/kg of body weight) per day.

Leptin: A hormone secreted by fat cells that has a central role in fat metabolism. Leptin was originally thought to be a signal to lose weight, but it may instead be a signal to the brain that there is fat in the body.

Lipids: Organic (carbon-containing) substances that do not dissolve in water. Lipids include fats, waxes, and related compounds.

Macronutrients: Nutrients in the diet that are the key sources of energy, namely protein, fat, and carbohydrates.

Meta-analysis: Process of using statistical methods to combine the results of different studies. A frequent application is pooling the results from a set of randomized controlled trials, none of which alone is powerful enough to demonstrate statistical significance.

Metabolic: Relating to metabolism, the whole range of biochemical processes that occur within living organisms. Metabolism consists of anabolism (the buildup of substances) and catabolism (the breakdown of substances). The term is commonly used to refer specifically to the breakdown of food and its transformation into energy.

Metabolic syndrome: A disorder characterized by a cluster of health problems, including increased waist circumference, high blood pressure, and abnormal lipid and blood sugar levels.

Microbiota: The microbiota is a large, complex, community of microorganisms that exist in a specific region—particularly in the digestive tracts of humans animals.

Normal weight: Ideal weight per height measurements; a classification of BMI between 18.5 and 24.9. Compared to overweight or obese, a body weight is less likely to be linked with any weight-related health problems, such as type 2 diabetes, heart disease, high blood pressure, and high blood cholesterol. A body mass index (BMI) of 18.5–24.9 is considered a healthy weight.

Nutrition: The process of the body using food to sustain life or the study of food and diet.

Obesity: An excessive amount of body fat in relation to lean body mass or a body weight that is 30 percent over the ideal weight for a specified height; BMI (body mass index) of 30 or greater.

Obesogenic: Environmental factors that may promote obesity and encourage the expression of a genetic predisposition to gain weight.

Orlistat: A lipase inhibitor used for weight loss. Lipase is an enzyme found in the bowel that assists in lipid absorption by the body. Orlistat blocks this enzyme, reducing the amount of fat the body absorbs by about 30 percent.

OTC: Over-the counter refers to nonprescription drugs.

Overweight: An excess of body weight but not necessarily body fat; a body mass index of 25–29.9 kilogram per square meter (kg/m2).

Pharmacotherapy: Treatment of disease through the use of drugs.

Phentermine: A drug used as an anorexic.

Prevalence: The total number of cases of a disease in a given population at a specific time.

Protein: One of the three nutrients that provides calories to the body. Protein is an essential nutrient that helps build many parts of the body, including muscle, bone, skin, and blood. Protein provides four calories per gram and is found in foods like meat, fish, poultry, eggs, dairy products, beans, nuts, and tofu.

RCT: A randomized clinical trial is an experiment in which subjects are randomly allocated into groups to receive or not to receive an experimental prevention or therapeutic product. RCTs are generally regarded as the most scientifically rigorous method of hypothesis testing available.

RMR: Resting metabolic rate accounts for 65–75 percent of daily energy expenditure and represents the minimum energy needed to maintain all physiological cell functions in the resting state. The principal determinant of RMR is lean body mass.

Satiation: Feeling of fullness that controls the meal size and duration.

Satiety: Quality or state of being fed or gratified to or beyond capacity.

Sedentary: Having low activity or exercise levels.

Sibutramine: A drug used for management of obesity that helps reduce food intake.

SSRI: Selective serotonin reuptake inhibitor is a neurochemical that enhances satisfaction from eating.

Systolic blood pressure: The maximum pressure in the artery produced as the heart contracts and blood begins to flow.

Type 2 diabetes: The most common form of diabetes, which occurs when the body is resistant to the action of insulin and the pancreas cannot make sufficient insulin to overcome this resistance; can be associated with obesity.

Underwater weighing: A method for determining body composition. It is also called hydrostatic weighing.

VLCD: A very low-calorie diet is a doctor-supervised diet that typically uses commercially prepared formulas to promote rapid weight loss in patients who are moderately to extremely obese. People on a VLCD consume about 800 calories per day or less.

Index

Note: Page numbers in *italics* followed by *p* indicate photographs, by *f* indicate figures, and by *t* indicate tables.

About the Authors

Alexandra Kazaks, Ph.D., RDN, CDE, is a professor at Bastyr University, Seattle, Washington. She received a doctorate in Nutritional Biology from the University of California, Davis. Her research has extended to magnesium and asthma management, the effects of plant-based foods on weight management and vascular disease risk factors, dietary supplements, and micronutrients. Her published works include ABC-CLIO's *Obesity: A Reference Handbook* (2009) and numerous journal articles, book chapters, and books. Dr. Kazaks is an active member of the Academy of Nutrition and Dietetics, American Association of Diabetes Educators, American Society of Nutrition, Institute of Food Technologists, and is a fellow of the Obesity Society.

Judith S. Stern, Sc.D., RDN has a degree from Cornell University and a doctorate from the Harvard School of Public Health where she studied with Dr. Jean Mayer, a leading researcher in obesity. She is a distinguished professor emeritus in the Departments of Nutrition and Internal Medicine and has published over 270 papers in scientific journals and several books (*How to Stay Slim and Health on the Fast Food Diet*, 1980; *Weighing the Options*, 1995; and *Obesity: A Reference Handbook*, 2009). She is a leader in professional societies and was president and co-founder of The Obesity Society. She was a contributing editor and columnist for *Vogue* magazine and wrote over 175 popular articles. Some of her honors include New York State 4-H Community Service State Winner, Institute of Medicine member, and along with Dr. Richard L. Atkinson, the first corecipient of the Atkinson-Stern Award for Distinguished Public Service from The Obesity Society.